Handbook of
PERIODONTOLOGY

Handbook of PERIODONTOLOGY

Satish Doiphode
BDS, MDS (Periodontology)

Ex-Professor
Government Dental College and Hospital
Aurangabad

Vaishali Ashtaputre
BDS, MDS (Periodontology)

Ex-Professor and Head
Department of Periodontology
CSMSS Dental College and Hospital
Aurangabad

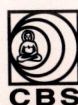

CBS

CBS Publishers & Distributors Pvt Ltd

New Delhi • Bengaluru • Chennai • Kochi • Kolkata • Mumbai
Hyderabad • Nagpur • Patna • Pune • Vijayawada

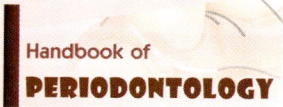

Handbook of
PERIODONTOLOGY

ISBN: 978-81-239-2853-1

First Edition: **2016**

Published by Satish Kumar Jain and produced by Varun Jain for
CBS Publishers & Distributors Pvt Ltd
4819/XI Prahlad Street, 24 Ansari Road, Daryaganj, New Delhi 110 002, India.
Ph: 23289259, 23266861, 23266867   Fax: 011-23243014
Website: www.cbspd.com   e-mail: delhi@cbspd.com; cbspubs@airtelmail.in.
Corporate Office: 204 FIE, Industrial Area, Patparganj, Delhi 110 092
Ph: 4934 4934   Fax: 4934 4935   e-mail: publishing@cbspd.com;
                                              publicity@cbspd.com

Branches

- **Bengaluru:** Seema House 2975, 17th Cross, K.R. Road, Banasankari 2nd Stage, Bengaluru 560 070, Karnataka
  Ph: +91-80-26771678/79   Fax: +91-80-26771680   e-mail: bangalore@cbspd.com
- **Chennai:** 7, Subbaraya Street, Shenoy Nagar, Chennai 600 030, Tamil Nadu
  Ph: +91-44-26680620, 26681266   Fax: +91-44-42032115   e-mail: chennai@cbspd.com
- **Kochi:** Ashana House, 39/1904, AM Thomas Road, Valanjambalam, Eranakulam 682 018, Kochi, Kerala
  Ph: +91-484-4059061-62-64-65   Fax: +91-484-4059065   e-mail: kochi@cbspd.com
- **Kolkata:** No. 6/B, Ground Floor, Rameswar Shaw Road, Kolkata 700 014, West Bengal
  Ph: +91-33-2289-1126, 1127, 1128,   e-mail: Kolkata@cbspd.com
- **Mumbai:** 83-C, Dr E Moses Road, Worli, Mumbai-400018, Maharashtra
  Ph: +91-22-24902340/41   Fax: +91-22-24902342   e-mail: mumbai@cbspd.com

Representatives

- **Hyderabad**   0-9885175004
- **Pune**   0-9623451994
- **Vijayawada** 0-9000660880
- **Nagpur**   0-9021734563
- **Patna**   0-9334159340

Printed at: Magic International, Greater Noida, UP

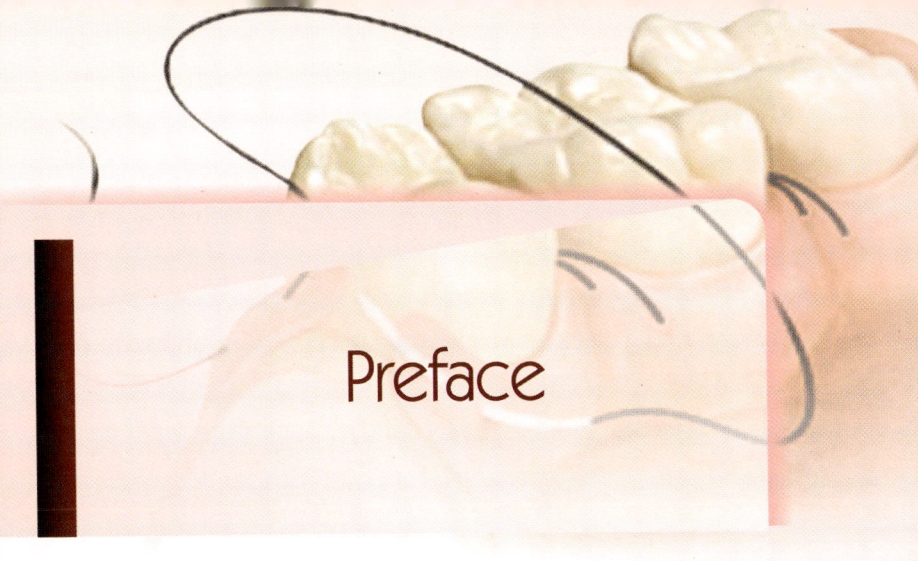

Preface

Periodontology provides the knowledge of tooth supporting structures. Preparation of the examination in this subject for undergraduate students is becoming increasingly important. Our experience in teaching has always demanded a concise material in periodontology from examination point of view.

This book is designed with the sole purpose of providing selective and precise coverage of the subject. The book has four main chapters which include definitions, compositions, differences and short notes, covering most of the DCI syllabus. It will be helpful for the students to revise the topics of the periodontology, especially during the theory and practical examinations and will be 'ready-reckoner' after going through the textbook of the subject.

The book is meant mainly for the undergraduate dental students. However, postgraduate students of periodontology as well as students of 'dental hygiene' and 'dental assisting' courses will also be benefited. Because of its concise nature, it can even prove to be valuable to the candidates preparing for postgraduate entrance examinations.

We are indebted to many of our colleagues who have helped us with valuable comments and suggestions. We express our sincere gratitude to Mr Dahale for typing the text and Mr Narendra Bhale for diagrams—we are extremely grateful for their wholehearted cooperation.

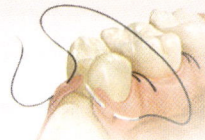

Mr K Ramesh of CBS Publishers & Distributors Pvt Ltd, Mumbai branch, requires a special mention here. We are also thankful to Mr YN Arjuna to provide us all the technical details.

Lastly, we would also like to thank our family members for their constant moral support and encouragement.

Satish Doiphode

Vaishali Ashtaputre

Contents

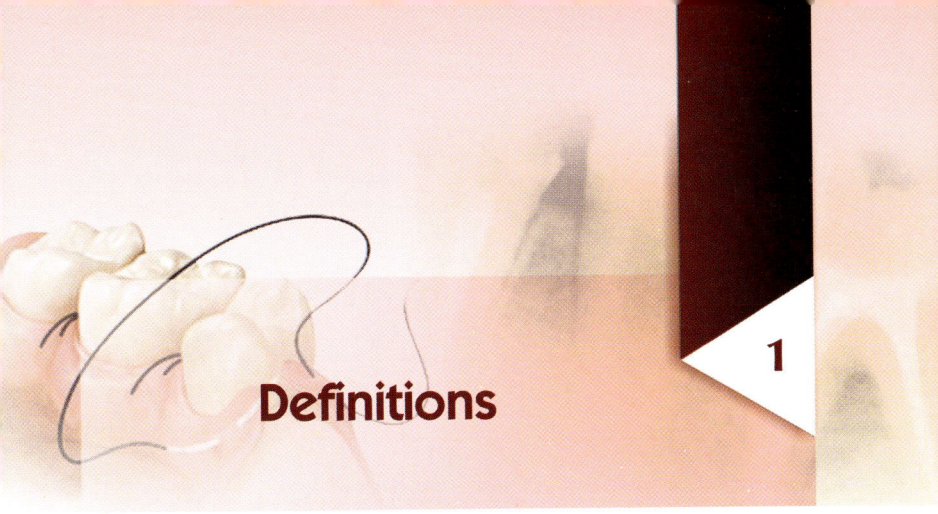

Definitions

DEFINITIONS

1. **Periodontia:** A branch of dentistry which deals with the structures around the tooth.
   Greek word   • *Peri*   –   around
              • *Odont*   –   tooth

2. **Periodontology:** The clinical science and study of periodontium (i.e. supporting structures of the tooth) in health and disease.

3. **Periodontics:** The practice of periodontology is periodontics (treatment part). It is the knowledge to treat periodontal diseases.

4. **Periodontium:** Supporting structures of the tooth, viz. gingiva, periodontal ligament, cementum, and alveolar bone (collective term).

5. **Oral mucous membrane:** Soft tissue membrane lining of the oral cavity. It may be classified into three different types—gingiva and the covering of the hard palate (masticatory mucosa), dorsum of the tongue (specialized mucosa), and the remainder of the oral mucous membrane (lining mucosa).

6. **Gingiva:** It is the part of masticatory mucosa that covers alveolar processes of the jaws and surrounds the necks of the teeth (*Carranza*).

7. **Junctional epithelium:** Collar-like band consisting of 10 to 20 layers thick stratified squamous non-keratinizing epithelium, 0.25 to 1.35 mm in length, attached to tooth

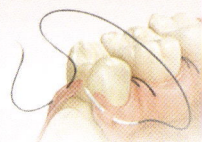

surface (epithelial attachment) by means of an internal basal lamina.

8. **Dentogingival unit:** It is a functional unit consisting of junctional epithelium and gingival fibers.

9. **Gingival sulcus:** It is a shallow, V-shaped space or crevice between tooth and free marginal gingiva. Its depth varies from 2 to 3 mm in clinically normal conditions.

10. **Periodontal ligament:** It is a connective tissue structure that surrounds the root of the tooth and connects it with the alveolar bone. (*Carranza*)

11. **Cementum:** It is a calcified, avascular mesenchymal tissue that forms the outer covering of the anatomic root. (*Carranza*)

12. **Alveolar bone (process):** Part of the maxilla and the mandible that forms and supports the tooth sockets. It develops with the eruption of the teeth and resorbs when the teeth are lost. (*Lindhe)*

13. **Aging:** It is a slowing down of natural function. It is between the physiological time related changes and the environmental pathological changes.

14. **Atrophy:** It is a decrease in the size of a normally developed cell, tissue, organ or part of the body after having come to full functional maturity. **OR** Exposure of the tooth by the apical migration of the gingiva is called gingival atrophy or gingival recession.

15. **Dystrophy:** Disorder resulting from defective or faulty cellular nutrition. The disturbances in cell metabolism are manifested by atrophy, degeneration, hyperplasia, as opposed to inflammation.

16. **Hyperplasia:** It is the increase in volume/size of a tissue, or organ caused by the abnormal multiplication or increase in the number of cells, which does not serve a functional purpose.

17. **Hypertrophy:** It is the increase in volume size of a tissue or organ produced entirely by the enlargement of existing cells in response to increased function.

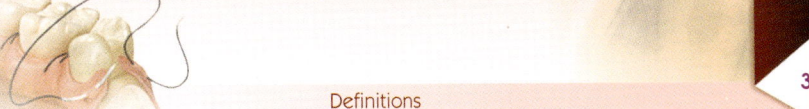
18. **Gingival recession:** It is the exposure of the root surface by an apical shift or the movement in the position of the gingiva. *(Grant)*

19. **Periodontal abscess:** Localized inflammatory lesion consisting of purulent material, i.e. collection of pus in periodontal tissues, or in a cavity formed by the disintegration of tissues, in which drainage is impaired.

20. **Periapical abscess:** Localized suppurative inflammation of tissues around the apex of the root of a tooth.

21. **Pericoronitis:** Inflammation of the soft tissues around a partially erupted tooth. It is mostly plaque associated and often aggravated by trauma from the tooth in opposing jaw.

22. **Inflammation:** It may be defined as the response of living tissue to a sublethal injury characterized by specific physiological and biochemical alterations.

23. **Bacteremia:** Presence of bacteria in the blood.

24. **Septicemia:** Morbid condition caused by the presence of pathogenic bacteria and their associated poisons in the blood.

25. **Collagen:** Fibrous insoluble protein found in the connective tissue including skin, bone, ligaments and cartilage.

26. **Crevicular fluid (gingival fluid):** Inflammatory products secreted from gingival vessels exhibiting pathologically increased permeability, related via gingival sulcus or pocket. Gingival fluid is considered as an inflammatory exudate, not a continuous transudate. *(Periodontal Literature review)*

27. **Intermediate plexus:** Central zone of periodontal ligament fibers, instead of being continuous the individual fiber consists of two separate parts spliced together midway between cementum and bone (Its existence is questionable.) *(Glickman)*

28. **Gingivitis:** Non-specific term used to denote inflammatory condition of gingiva, regardless of the etiology, which is progressive and reversible.

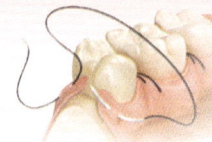

29. **Diffuse gingivitis:** Inflammatory condition of gingiva involving the marginal, papillary and attached gingiva (collective term).

30. **Desmosomes:** Structures that join epithelial cells together, which are composed of adjacent cell membranes and a pair of attachment plaques as well as intervening extracellular structures.

31. **Periodontitis:** It is a generalized term used to connote inflammation of the periodontium (i.e. gingiva, periodontal ligament, cementum and alveolar bone.)

32. **Chronic periodontitis:** In this the progressive destruction of periodontal tissues mainly associated with specific microbial plaque induced inflammation, clinically resulting into pocket formation, recession or both.

33. **Periodontitis associated with trauma from occlusion (TFO):** This term is used to denote chronic periodontitis when associated with occlusal trauma. (Old term: Compound periodontitis)

34. **Aggressive periodontitis:** It is characterized by rapid rate of disease progression of periodontium seen in an otherwise healthy individual where the amount of destruction does not commensurate with the amount of local irritants; with the history suggestive of genetic trait.

    It can be localized or generalized.

35. **Localized aggressive periodontitis (LAP):** It is characterized as having localized first molar/incisor involvement with interproximal attachment loss on at least two permanent teeth, one of which is first molar and involving no more than two teeth other than first molars and incisors. (*Carranza*)

36. **Diagnosis:** It is knowledge and identity of a condition, entity or a syndrome. It's an art of identifying or recognizing disease.

37. **Desquamative gingivitis (gingivosis):** Uncommon gingivitis characterized by intense redness, desquamation and ulceration of surface epithelium. (*Prinz*)

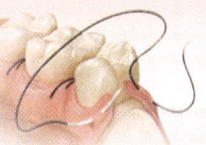

38. **Ulcer:** Break in the continuity of the lining of a mucous membrane/epithelium (surface), produced by sloughing of necrotic inflammatory tissue.

39. **Epidemiology:** It is the study of the distribution and determinants of health-related states or events in specified populations, and the application of this study to control health problems. *(Last JM)*

40. **Acute necrotizing ulcerative gingivitis (ANUG):** (Vincent's disease): Acute inflammatory destructive disease of the gingiva characterized by necrosis and ulceration of the surface of the gingiva with punched-out crater-like depression at the crest of the interdental gingiva.

41. **Prognosis:** The prognosis is a prediction of the duration, course and termination of a disease and its response to treatment. *(Periodontal literature review)*

42. **Treatment plan:** The treatment plan is the scheduled sequence of therapeutic measures used to cure or treat the patient's periodontal disease. (The treatment plan is the blue-print for case management.)

43. **Splint:** Device or appliance used to stabilize mobile teeth and redistribute occlusal forces.

44. **Stippling:** It is a orange peel-pitted appearance of the attached gingiva and central part of the interdental gingiva.

45. **Stillman's cleft:** Defect or apostrophe-shaped indentations extending from and into the gingival margin for varying distance usually on the facial surface. (Specific type of gingival recession)

46. **McCall festoons:** These are life-saver shaped enlargements or rolled out thickened band of the marginal gingiva that occur most frequently in the canine and premolar areas on the facial surface.

47. **Dehiscence:** This is the bony defect in which the root is denuded of bone, extending from marginal bone for a variable distance, and is covered only by periosteum and overlying gingiva.

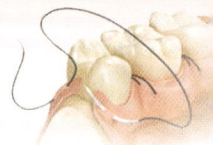

48. **Fenestration:** Isolated area in which the root is denuded of bone and the root surface is covered only be periosteum and overlying gingiva. Here the marginal bone is intact. *(Grat, Stern, Listgarten)*

49. **Gingival fibers:** The connective tissue of the marginal gingiva is densely collagenous, containing prominent system of collagen fiber bundles which are known as gingival fibers. *(Carranza)*

50. **Pocket:** Pathological deepening of gingival sulcus. *(Carranza)*

51. **Subgingival curettage:** It is a procedure that is performed apical to the epithelial attachment, severing the connective tissue attachment down to the osseous crest. *(Carranza)*

52. **Gingivectomy:** It is the excision of the diseased soft tissue wall of the periodontal pocket with thorough smoothening of the roots.

53. **Gingivoplasty:** It is the re-contouring of the gingiva which has lost its physiological contour (form), in the absence of periodontal pocket. *(Carranza)*

54. **Periodontal flap:** It is a section of gingiva and/or mucosa surgically separated from the underlying tissues to provide visibility of, and access to the underlying periodontal structures, i.e. bone and root surface. *(Carranza)*

55. **Trauma from occlusion:** When occlusal forces exceed the adaptive capacity of the tissues, tissue injury results. The resultant injury is termed trauma from occlusion. *(Orban)*

    • It is the tissue injury and not the occlusal force.

56. **Periodontal plastic surgery** (mucogingival surgery)**:** It consists of plastic surgical procedures for the correction of gingiva–mucous membrane relationships that complicate periodontal disease and may interfere with the success of periodontal treatment. (*American Academy of Periodontology, World workshop, 1996*)

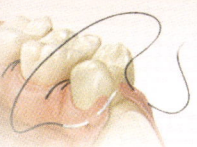

57. **Furcation involvement:** The conditions in which the bifurcation and trifurcation of multi-rooted teeth are denuded by periodontal disease.

58. **Graft:** A graft is viable tissue that, after removal from a donor site, is implanted within a host tissue which is then restored, repaired or regenerated.

59. **Osseous surgery:** The procedure by which changes in the alveolar bone can be accomplished to rid it of deformities induced by the periodontal disease. *(Carranza)*

60. **Frenectomy:** It is the complete removal of the frenum, including its attachment to the underlying alveolar process.

61. **Frenotomy:** It is the simple incisional release of the frenum from its insertion to its base.

62. **Osteoplasty:** It is a plastic surgical procedure by which non-tooth supporting bone is reshaped to achieve a physiological gingival and osseous contour for the purpose of pocket elimination in areas of tori, exostoses, thick bony margins, blunted interdental septa, etc.

63. **Ostectomy:** It is the plastic surgical procedure by which radicular and interradicular tooth supporting bone is removed to eliminate deformities.

64. **Microbial plaque:** It is a complex, tenaciously attached soft deposit composed of organized structure of micro-organisms, epithelial cells, leukocytes, and macrophages in an inter-microbial matrix.

65. **Dental plaque:** It is defined clinically as a structured resilient, yellow, grayish substance consists mainly of microorganisms that adhere tenaciously to the teeth and removable or fixed restorations. *(Bowen)*

66. a. **Bruxism:** Habitual grinding of the teeth specifically when the individual is not chewing or swallowing.

    b. **Clenching:** In which a person holds the teeth firmly together with force. *(Carranza)*

67. **Calculus:** It is mineralized microbial plaque attached to natural teeth and dental prosthesis.

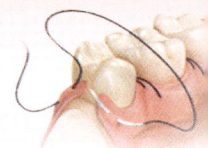

68. **Col:** A valley-like depression that connects the facial and lingual tips of the papillae and conforms to the shape of the interproximal contact *(Cohen)*

69. **Xeroradiography:** This is a process by which X-ray images are recorded by means of a xerographic copying method. It does not involve wet chemical processing or the use of a dark room.

70. **Xenografts:** A tissue graft transplanted from a donor of a different species than the host.

71. **General adaptation syndrome (GAS):** The cumulative systemic reactions that result from continued exposure to stress is termed as general adaptation syndrome. *(Selye)*

72. **Repair:** Repair simply restores the continuity of diseased marginal gingiva and reestablishes a normal gingival sulcus at the same level on the root as the base of the preexisting periodontal pocket (Tissue heals by scar). *(Carranza)*

73. **Regeneration:** It is the growth and differentiation of new cells and intercellular substances to form new tissues. It is a renewal of structures). *(Carranza)*

74. **New attachment:** It is the embedding of new periodontal ligament fibers into new cementum and thus forming the new attachment of gingival epithelium to a tooth surface previously denuded by disease. *(Carranza)*

75. **Epithelial adaptation:** It is a close apposition of the gingival epithelium to the tooth surface, with no gain in the height of gingival fiber attachment. *(Carranza)*

76. **Reattachment:** It refers to repair in areas of the root not previously exposed to the pocket, such as after surgical detachment of the tissues or following tears in the cementum, tooth fractures, etc. *(Carranza)*

77. **Halitosis:** Unpleasant foul breath arising from odors that are emitted from the oral cavity.

78. **Food impaction:** Forceful wedging of food into the periodontium by altered occlusal forces. *(Carranza)*

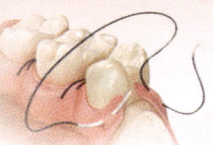

79. **Plunger cusps:** Cusps that tend to wedge food forcibly into interproximal embrasure spaces are known as plunger cusps. *(Carranza)*

80. **Attrition:** It is occlusal wear resulting from functional contacts with opposing teeth. *(Carranza)*

81. **Facets:** The occlusal or incisal surfaces worn by attrition are called facets, which are smooth and shiny.

82. **Abrasion:** It is the abnormal wearing away of tooth structure/substance due to mechanical process, other than that of mastication.

83. **Erosion:** It is a sharply defined, wedge-shaped depression in the cervical areas of the facial tooth surface, usually caused due to chemicals. *(Carranza)*

84. **Abfraction:** Tooth wear resulting from occlusal loading surfaces causing tooth flexure and mechanical micro-fractures and tooth substance loss in the cervical area. *(Carranza)*

85. **Embrasures:** When adjacent teeth are in contact, the spaces that widen out from the contact are known as embrasures. It is the interproximal space beneath the area of tooth contact. *(Carranza)*

86. **Reverse architecture of bone:** It is the resorption of bone when there is more rapid rate of resorption of the interproximal bone including facial and lingual plates than radiculer bone of a tooth, thereby reversing the normal architecture.

87. **Gingival pocket (pseudopocket):** It is formed by gingival enlargement without destruction of the underlying periodontal tissues. *(Carranza)*

88. **Periodontal pocket (true pocket):** It is the pathological deepening of the gingival sulcus which leads to destruction of the supporting periodontal tissues and loosening and exfoliation of the teeth. *(Carranza)*

89. **Suprabony pockets:** In this, the bottom of the periodontal pocket is coronal to the underlying alveolar bone. *(Carranza)*

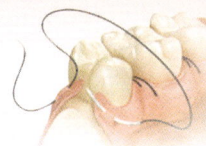

90. **Infrabony pocket (intrabony)** (subcrestal or intra-alveolar): In this, the bottom of the pocket is apical to the level of the adjacent alveolar bone. (*Carranza*)

91. **Scaling:** It is the procedure by which plaque and calculus are removed from both supragingival and subgingival tooth surfaces.

92. **Root planing:** It is the procedure by which residual embedded calculus and portions of cementum are removed from the roots to produce a smooth, hard and clean surface. (*Carranza*)

93. **Oral prophylaxis:** It is a scaling and polishing performed on dental patients in good periodontal health to remove supragingival plaque, stain, and deposits to prevent caries and periodontal disease.

94. **Oral physiotherapy:** Those procedures practiced by a patient for the purpose of maintaining good oral hygiene. (*Glickman*)

95. **Oral hygiene:** Science of cleanliness of oral cavity.

96. **Coronoplasty:** It is the selective reduction of areas on occlusal surface with the primary aim of creating the mechanical conditions in contact situations and the neural pattern of sensory input.

97. **Combined osseous defect:** When the number of walls in the apical portion of the defect (osseous) are greater than that in its coronal portion the term combined osseous defect is used.

98. **Granuloma pyogenicum:** It is a tumor-like gingival enlargement considered to be an exaggerated conditioned response to minor trauma.

99. **Electrosurgery:** This is surgical technique performed on soft tissues by using controlled high frequency electrical current in the range of 1.5 to 7.5 million cycles/second.

100. **Ultrasonic:** The term ultrasonic is defined as pertaining to mechanical radiant energy having a frequency beyond the upper limit of perception by the human ear, that is beyond 20,000 cycles/second.

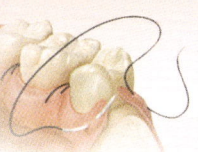

101. AIDS: Stands for acquired immune deficiency syndrome caused by human immunodeficiency virus (HIV) and characterized by profound impairment of the immune system.

102. Cryosurgery: It offers a means of destroying tissues by subjecting it to extreme cold.

103. Materia alba: Bacteria and their product mixed with exfoliated epithelial cells, leukocytes, and food debris may form loose deposits overlying tooth surfaces, which do not possess the structural organization of plaque, is termed as materia alba.

104. Communicable disease: It signifies a capacity for the maintenance of infection by natural modes of spread, such as direct contact through drinking water, food, and eating utensils, via the airborne route.

105. Transmissible: It represents a capacity for the maintenance of an infectious agent in successive passages through a susceptible animal host.

106. Motivation: It is the responsibility of instructor to bridge the gap between the patient's needs and the instructional goals.

107. Dental implant: A device implanted into the oral tissues beneath the mucosa, periosteum and/or within the bone to provide retention and support for a prosthesis.

108. Osseointegration: It is defined as the direct structural and functional connection between ordered, living bone and the surface of a load carrying implant. *(Branemark)*

109. Peri-implantitis: It is the progressive peri-implant bone loss in conjunction with a soft tissue inflammatory lesion.

110. Peri-implant mucositis: Inflammatory changes which are confined to the soft tissue surrounding an implant are diagnosed as peri-implant mucositis. *(Carranza)*

111. Growth factors: Growth factors are polypeptide molecules, released by cells in inflamed area, that regulate events in wound healing. *(Carranza)*

112. Epidemiological Index: It is a data collection tool that aid in measurement and evaluation of disease indicators and

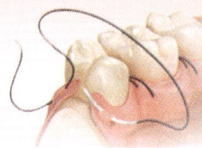

conditions, classification systems featuring numbered scales against which a specific population may be compared. **OR** Epidemiological indices attempt to quantitate clinical conditions on the graduated scale.

113. **Dental epidemiology:** It is the study of the pattern, distribution and dynamics of dental diseases in human population, and application of this study to control dental health problems. (*Last*)

114. **Prevalence:** Prevalence is the proportion of persons affected by a disease (**old and new both**) at a specific point in time as determined by cross-sectional survey.

115. **Incidence:** Incidence is defined as the rate of occurrence of **new** disease in a population during a given interval of time.

116. **Refractory periodontitis:** Cases of periodontitis that for unknown reason do not respond to therapy and/or recur soon after adequate treatment have been referred to as refractory periodontitis. (*American Academy of Periodontology*)

117. **Osteoconduction:** Osteoconduction is a physical process in which the graft material acts as scaffolding for new bone to cover over.

118. **Osteoinduction:** Osteoinduction is a chemical process by which the graft material is capable of promoting and converting neighboring cells into osteoblasts, which in turn form bone.

119. **Guided bone regeneration (GBR):** Guided bone regeneration is the term used for regeneration of bone defects in implant surgery.

120. **Microsurgery:** Microsurgery may be defined as a refinement in operative technique by which visual acuity is improved through magnification. (*Carranza*)

121. **Virulence factors:** The properties that enable a bacterium to cause disease are termed as virulence factors.

122. **Necrotizing ulcerative progressive periodontitis (NUP):** It is a severe and rapidly progressive disease that has a distinctive erythema necrosis and ulceration of the free

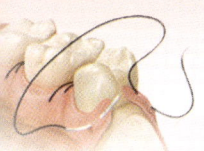

gingiva, attached gingiva and alveolar mucosa and severe bone loss. It is an eaxtension of necrotizing ulcerative gingivitis into periodontium leading to bone loss.

123. **Guided tissue regeneration (GTR):** It is a technique used for prevention of migration of epithelial cells and repopulation of desired cells.

124. **Antigen:** A toxin or other foreign substance which induces an immune response in the body, especially the production of antibodies.

125. **Antibody:** An immunoglobuline produced by B cells that is used by immune system to identify and neutralize the antigen.

126. **Antioxident:** It is a substance which slows down the damage that can be caused to other substances by the effects of oxygen.

127. **Antibiotics:** These are the medicinal substances, produced from micro-organisms and capable of killing the bacteria or slowing their growth.

128. **Probiotics:** These are the micro-organisms that have claimed health benefits when consumed, e.g. *Lactobacillus.*

129. **Antimicrobials:** Chemical substances synthetically prepared to treat the microbial infection.

130. **Analgesics:** Medications that reduce or eliminate pain.

131. **Anti-inflammatory:** The property of the drug or treatment that counteracts or suppresses inflammation.

132. **Gingival zenith:** Marginal gingiva is generally scalloped. The height of convexity of scalloping is called 'gingival zenith'.

Producing esthetically pleasing gingival zenith is key factor in cosmetic dentistry. (*Carranza*)

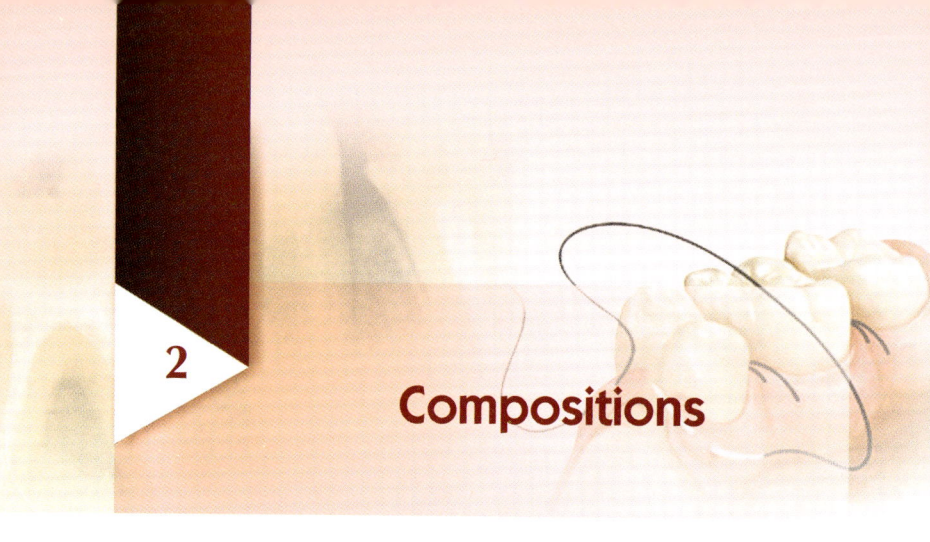

2 Compositions

1. GINGIVAL SULCULAR FLUID

a. Cellular elements

1. Polymorphonuclear neutrophils (PMNs)
2. Lymphocytes and monocytes
3. Desquamated epithelial cells
4. Bacteria

b. Electrolytes

1. Potassium
2. Sodium and calcium

c. Organic compounds

1. Carbohydrates
2. Proteins
3. Immunoglobulins—IgG, IgA, IgM.

d. Metabolic and bacterial products

1. Lactic acid
2. Urea
3. Hydroxyproline
4. Endotoxins
5. Cytotoxic substance
6. Hydrogen sulfide

e. Antibacterial factors

f. Several enzymes

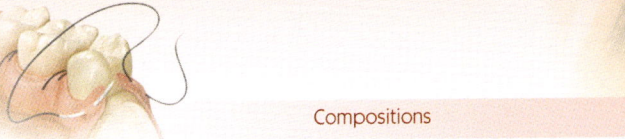

2. MICROBIAL PLAQUE

a. Microorganisms

1. Proliferating bacteria
2. Non-bacterial microorganisms
   a. Archaea
   b. Yeast
   c. Protozoa
   d. Viruses

b. Intercellular matrix

i. Host cells
   1. Epithelial cells
   2. Macrophages
   3. Leukocytes

ii. Organic components
   1. Polysaccharide
   2. Protein; glycoproteins
   3. Lipid material
   4. DNA and albumin

iii. Inorganic components
   1. Calcium
   2. Phosphorus
   3. Trace amounts of other minerals, such as sodium, potassium and fluoride

3. CALCULUS

a. Inorganic contents

1. Calcium phosphate—75.9%
2. Calcium carbonate—3.1%
3. Magnesium phosphate—traces

Principal inorganic components

1. Calcium—39%
2. Phosphorus—19%
3. Carbon dioxide—1.9%
4. Magnesium—0.8%

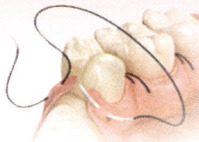

Trace amounts of sodium, zinc, strontium, bromine, silicon, iron and fluorine. Two-thirds of inorganic components are in form of crystals:

a. Hydroxyapatite—58% approximately
b. Octacalcium phosphate—12% approximately
c. Magnesium whitlockite—21% approximately
d. Brushite—9% approximately

b. Organic contents

a. Carbohydrate—1.9 to 9.1%
b. Protein—5.9 to 8.2%
c. Lipid—0.2%
d. Desquamated epithelial cells
e. Leukocytes
f. Various types of microorganisms.

4. DISCLOSING AGENTS

a. Basic fuchsin

1. Basic fuchsin—6 gm
2. Ethyl alcohol—95% 100 ml
   Add two drops to water in a dappen dish.

b. Potassium iodide

1. Iodine crystals—1.6 gm
2. Water—13.4 ml
3. Glycerin to make 30 ml

c. Wafers

FDC red (erythrosine)—15 gm
Sodium chloride—0.74%
Sodium sucaryl—0.74%
Calcium stearate—0.995%
Soluble saccharin—0.186%
White oil—0.124%

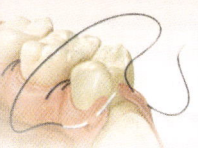

Flavoring agents (FDA approved)—2.239%

Sorbitol to make—7 grain wafer

(To be crushed between teeth and swished around the mouth for 30 seconds).

5. DESENSITIZING AGENTS

Agents used by Patient

Powder/Paste

1. Strontium chloride 10%/potassium nitrate 5%
2. Sodium monofluorophosphate 0.7%
3. Formaldehyde
4. Polyglycol

Agents used by the Dental Surgeon in the clinic

a. Zinc chloride 8 to 12%

b. Strontium chloride 10%

Other Agents

Silver nitrate (nostrum)

Sodium fluoride, kaolin, glycerin in paste form

Corticosteroids

Iontophoresis

Restorative resins

Dentin bonding agents

Cavity varnishes

Anti-inflammatory agents

6. PERIODONTAL DRESSING

1. Zinc oxide–eugenol dressing

  a. Powder

Zinc oxide	43.5%
Rosin	45.0%
Kaolin	3.0%
Fine asbestos fibers (Binder and filler)	4.0%

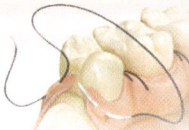

| Zinc acetate (Accelerator) | 1.5% |

b. Liquid

Eugenol	85%
Cotton seed oil (Added to dissolve eugenol)	14.%
Thymol	1.0%

2. Non-eugenol dressing: Powder and liquid

a. Powder

Rosin	0.52 gm
Zinc oxide	0.41 gm
Bacitracin	3000 units

b. Liquid (ointment)

| Zinc oxide | 5% |
| Hydrogenated fat | 95% |

3. Non-eugenol dressing: Paste form (**Coe-Pak**)

a. Tube 1 paste
   1. Metallic oxide (zinc oxide)
   2. Oil for plasticity
   3. Gum for cohesiveness
   4. Lorothidol—fungicide

b. Tube 2
   1. Coconut fatty acids thickened with colophony resin (Rosin)
   2. Chlorothymol—bacteriostatic

4. Cyanoacrylates—N–butyl cyanoacrylate

5. Tissue conditioners
   – Methacrylic gels
   – Antibacterial agents.

7. POVIDONE IODINE

a. Solution	5–10%
b. Surgical scrub	7.5%
c. Spray	5.%

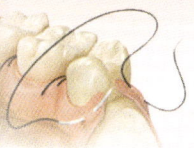

8. POLISHING PASTE

Pumice powder   –   Abrasive agent
Glycerin   –   Vehicle
Flavoring agents can be added
Various polishing pastes are available in the market.

9. GUM PAINT

Glycerol	72%
Iodine	0.03%
Menthol	0.05%
Potassium iodide	0.05%
Tannic acid	
Thymol	0.033%

Various gum paints are available in the market.

10. DENTIFRICES

1. **Abrasive agent (20–40%):** Used as cleaning and polishing agent—silica, phosphate salts, carbonates
2. **Binder (11%):** Used as stabilizer
   Natural: Carboxymethylcellulose (CMC)
   Synthetic: Polymers
3. **Humectant (48–60%):** Prevents loss of water—glycerin, sorbitol, polyethylene glycol, xylitol, propylene glycol
4. **Sweetener (0.20%):** Saccharin
5. **Flavor (1%):** Improves taste—minty, fruity, salty, medicinal, cinnamon
6. **Surfactant (1.7%):** Foaming agent enables debris removal—sodium lauryl sulfate
7. **Active agents:**
   a. **Fluoride (0.82%):** Anticariogenic—sodium-monofluoro-phosphate, stannous fluoride
   b. **Antitartar (0.2%):** Polyphosphates, zinc citrate
   c. **Antiplaque (0.2%):** Triclosan

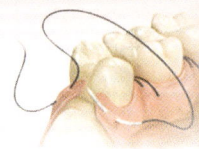

d. **Desensitizing agent (5%):** Potassium nitrate

e. **Whitening agent (0.5%):** Calcium peroxide, hydrogen peroxide

f. **Coloring agent (0.05%)**

g. **Water:** To make 100%

11. STIMULANT MIXTURE

1. Spirit of ether 2.5 cc (pharmaceutical aid)

2. Spirit aromatic ammonia 10.5 cc
   (Stimulant and antidepressant)

3. Spirit chloroform 2.5 cc
   Add water to make it 100 cc

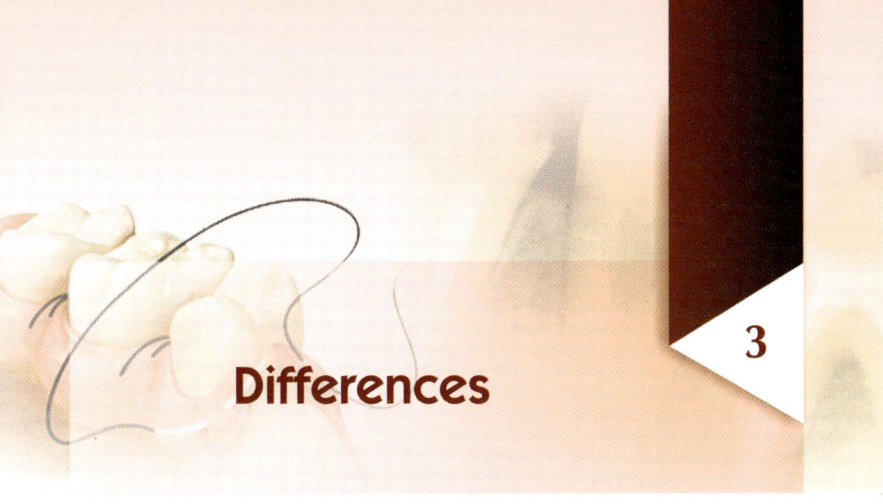

Differences

3

1. Supragingival and subgingival calculus

Supragingival calculus	Subgingival calculus
1. Refers to calculus coronal to the marginal gingiva.	Refers to calculus below the crest of the marginal gingiva.
2. It is visible in the oral cavity.	It is not visible on routine oral examination
3. It is termed as salivary calculus—derived from saliva	It is termed as serumal calculus—derived from blood serum (gingival fluid).
4. It is usually white or whitish yellow in color.	It is usually dark brown or greenish black.
5. It has a clay-like consistency and is easily detached from the tooth surface.	It has a flint-like hard consistency and is firmly attached to the tooth surface.
6. It consists of hydroxyapatite, magnesium whitlockite, octacalcium phosphate and brushite crystals.	It has the same hydroxyapatite content more magnesium whitlockite and less brushite and octacalcium phosphate crystals.
7. The morphological different forms may not be present.	The following forms have been described. a. Crusty, spiny, or nodular type. b. Ring-like or ledge-like encircling the tooth

Contd.

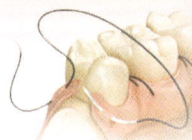

Contd.

Supragingival calculus	Subgingival calculus
	c. Veneer type consisting of a thin, glassy, smooth layer.
	d. Finger-like or fern-like extensions toward the bottom of the periodontal pocket.
	e. Individual islands or spots of calculus. Combination of these forms may occur.
8. In presence of supragingival calculus, periodontal pocket may not be present.	Usually periodontal pocket present.

2. Periodontal and periapical abscesses

Periodontal abscess	Periapical abscess
1. It is a localized accumulation of pus within the gingival wall of a periodontal pocket (Fig. 3.2A).	It is a localized accumulation of pus, infective material, etc. around root tip (Fig. 3.1).
2. Tooth is tender on lateral percussion.	Tooth is tender on vertical percussion.
3. Vitality of tooth or teeth is present.	Tooth or teeth are non-vital.
4. In chronic periodontal abscess, the draining sinus is present at the gingival mucosa.	In chronic periapical abscess, the draining sinus is present at the alveolar mucosa.
5. History of long-standing pocket or periodontal disease present.	History of long-standing trauma or carious lesion present.
6. Radiographic appearance shows radiolucency along the lateral aspect of the tooth (In long-standing abscess).	Radiographic appearance shows radiolucency around the root tip (In long-standing injury)

Contd.

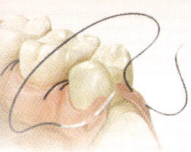

Contd.

Periodontal abscess	Periapical abscess
7. Chronic periodontal abscess does not cause change in color of the tooth.	Chronic periapical abscess may cause change in color of the tooth.
8. Swelling is present around the gingival zone of the involved tooth.	Swelling is present around the alveolar mucosa of the involved tooth.
9. It is acute exacerbations of periodontal disease.	It is a result of pulpal infection.
10. Pain usually dull and localized.	Pain often severe and difficult to localize.

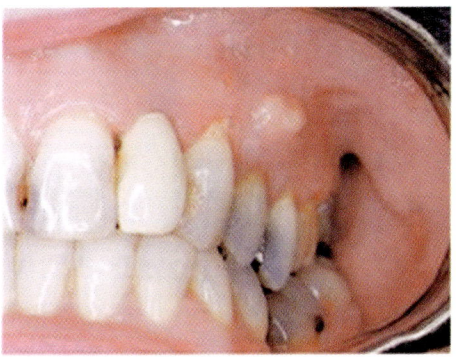

Fig. 3.1: Periapical abscess

3. Periodontal and gingival abscess

Periodontal abscess	Gingival abscess
1. The periodontal abscess involves the supporting periodontal structures (Fig. 3.2A).	The gingival abscess is confined to the marginal gingiva (Fig. 3.2B).
2. It generally occurs in the course of chronic destructive periodontitis.	It often occurs in previously disease-free areas

Contd.

Contd.

Periodontal abscess	Gingival abscess
3. Long-standing pathology is present.	It is usually an acute inflammatory response to forcing of foreign material into the gingiva.

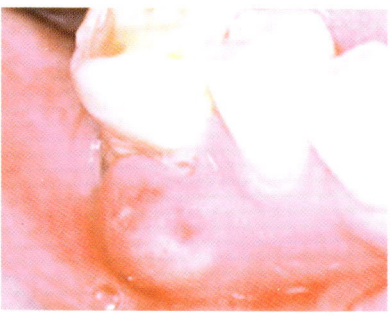

Fig. 3.2A: Periodontal abscess

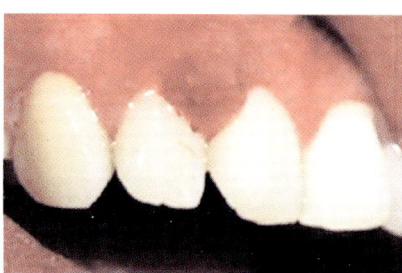

Fig. 3.2B: Gingival abscess

4. Suprabony and infrabony pockets

Suprabony pocket	Infrabony pocket
1. The base of the pocket is coronal to the level of the alveolar bone.	The base of the pocket is apical to the crest of the alveolar bone
2. The pattern of destruction of the underlying bone is horizontal.	The pattern of destruction of the underlying bone or adjacent bone is vertical.

Contd.

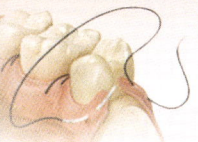

Contd.

Suprabony pocket	Infrabony pocket
3. On the facial and lingual surfaces, the periodontal ligament fibers beneath the pocket follow their normal horizontal oblique course between the tooth and the bone.	On the facial and lingual surfaces, the periodontal ligament fibers follow the angular pattern of the adjacent bone. They extend from the cementum beneath the base of the pocket along the bone and cover the crest to join with the outer periosteum.
4. Interproximally, the transseptal fibers that are restored during progressive periodontal disease are arranged horizontally in the space between the base of the pocket and the alveolar bone.	Interproximally, the transseptal fibers are oblique rather than horizontal. They extend from the cementum beneath the base of the pocket along the bone and over the crest to the cementum of the adjacent tooth.
5. Formation of the suprabony pocket is due to long-standing inflammation due to microbial plaque	Formation of the infrabony pocket is due to long-standing inflammation and trauma from occlusion could be the aggravating factor.
6. There is overall generalized horizontal bone loss	There is affection of bony walls of the tooth in form of one-walled, two-walled and three-walled defect

5. Acute necrotizing ulcerative gingivitis and acute herpetic gingivostomatitis

Acute necrotizing ulcerative gingivitis	Acute herpetic gingivostomatitis
1. Etiology—interaction between host and bacteria mostly fusospirochetes.	Specific viral etiology.

Contd.

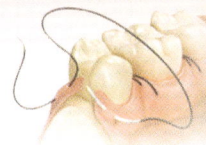

Contd.

Acute necrotizing ulcerative gingivitis	Acute herpetic gingivostomatitis
2. Necrotizing condition	Diffuse erythema and vesicular eruption
3. Punched out interdental gingival margin—pseudomembrane that peels off, leaving raw areas	Vesicles rupture and leave slightly depressed oval or spherical ulcer.
4. Marginal gingiva may get affected, other tissues rarely	Diffuse involvement or gingiva, may include buccal mucosa and lips
5. Deep ulcers	Shallow ulcers
6. Relatively uncommon in children.	Occurs more frequently in children.
7. No definite duration	Duration of 7–10 days
8. No demonstrated immunity	Presence of some degree of immunity
9. Contagion not demonstrated	Contagious.
10. Predisposing factors, such as poor oral hygiene, stress, nutritional deficiency, may be present.	No such factor.
11. Responds well to antibiotic and antimicrobial therapy, such as penicillin and metronidazole	No specific antibiotic therapy is proved.
12. If untreated (in some cases) may lead to Nom and death	Self-limiting condition

6. Gingivectomy and gingivoplasty

Gingivectomy	Gingivoplasty
1. It is the surgical excision of the diseased gingival tissue to reduce the depth of the periodontal pockets	It is the surgical reshaping and recontouring of the gingiva to produce physiologic contour.

Contd.

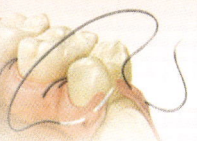

Gingivectomy	Gingivoplasty
2. Suprabony periodontal pockets present	Pseudo (gingival) pocket present

7. Ostectomy and osteoplasty

Ostectomy	Osteoplasty
It is the surgical removal of tooth supporting bone for the purpose of periodontal pocket elimination.	It is the surgical reshaping of non-tooth supporting bone around the tooth to produce physiological form

8. Frenectomy and frenotomy

Frenectomy	Frenotomy
It is complete removal of the frenum including its attachment to underlying bone.	It is the simple incisional release of the frenum from the apex of its insertioin to its base.

9. Atrophy and dystrophy

Atrophy	Dystrophy
Decrease in the size of a normally developed cell, tissue, organ after having come to full functional maturity.	Disorder resulting from defective or faulty cellular nutritioin.

10. Hypertrophy and hyperplasia

Hypertrophy	Hyperplasia
Increase in the volume of a tissue or organ produced entirely by the enlargement of existing cell. (Response to functional demands)	Increase in volume of a tissue or organ causd by the abnormal multiplication or increase in the number of cells (Does not serve a functional purpose)

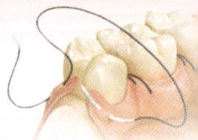

11. Hyperplastic gingivitis and gingival hyperplasia

Hyperplastic gingivitis	*Gingival hyperplasia*
It is the increase in size of the gingiva with enlargement produced due to inflammation. (Etiology is inflammation.)	It is the increase in size of the gingiva with enlargement produced in absence of inflammation. (Etiology is other than inflammation.)

12. Dehiscence and fenestration

Dehiscence	*Fenestration*
It is the bony defect in which the root is denuded of bone extending from marginal bone, for a variable distance, from the alveolar crest and the root surface is covered by periosteum and gingiva.	It is isolated area or a circumscribed window, in which the root is denuded of bone and does not communicate with the crestal margin and the root surface is covered only by periosteum and overlying gingiva. (Marginal bone is intact.)

13. Gingival recession and pocket formation

Gingival recession	*Pocket formation*
It is the exposure of root surface by an apical shift in the position of the gingiva	Pathological deepening of the sulcus is called as pocket formation

14. Bacteremia and septicemia

Bacteremia	*Septicemia*
Presence of bacteria in the blood	Presence of pathogenic bacteria and their associated toxins in the blood (Morbid condition)

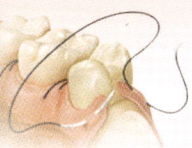

15. Acellular cementum and cellular cementum

Acellular cementum	Cellular cementum
1. Also called as primary cementum	Also called as secondary cementum
2. First to be formed	Formed after acellular cementum
3. Formed before the tooth reaches the occlusal plane.	Formed after the tooth reaches the occlusal plane
4. Covers the cervical third or half of the root	Covers the apical third of the root
5. More calcified	Less calcified
6. No cells are present	Cementocytes in lacunae connected by canaliculi are present.
7. Majority of the structure is made up of Sharpey's fiber	Less Sharpey's fiber content

16. Acute herpetic gingivostomatitis and aphthous stomatitis

Acute herpetic gingivostomatitis	Aphthous stomatitis
1. Cause—herpes simplex virus (HSV-1)	Unknown cause
2. Contagious	Non-contagious
3. Occurs on keratinized areas of oral cavity and oral mucosa	Occurs on non-keratinized areas of oral cavity
4. Occurs frequently in infants and children below 6 years of age	Occurs at any age
5. Diffuse erythema and vesicular eruption	Discrete spherical vesicles Saucer like, red or grayish central red portion and elevated rim at periphery
6. No different forms of herpes seen	Three different clinical forms present—minor, major and recurrent

Contd.

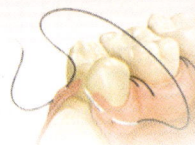

Contd.

Acute herpetic gingivostomatitis	Aphthous stomatitis
7. Not painful unless complicated	Very painful condition
8. Antiviral treatment can be done	No specific treatment

17. Acute necrotizing ulcerative gingivitis and desquamative gingivitis

Acute necrotizing ulcerative gingivitis	Desquamative gingivitis
1. Acute history	Chronic history
2. Painful	May/may not be painful
3. Marginal gingiva affected	Diffuse involvement of marginal and attached gingivae and other areas of oral mucosa
4. Pseudomembrane formation seen	Patchy desquamation of gingival epithelium
5. Papillary and marginal necrotic lesions	Papillae do not undergo necrosis
6. Characteristic fetid odor	None
7. Bacterial smears show fusospirochetal complex	Bacterial smears reveal numerous epithelial cells few bacterial forms
8. Affects adults of both sexes, occasionally children	Affects adults, most often women.

18. Attached gingiva and alveolar mucosa

Attached gingiva	Alveolar mucosa
1. Keratinized	Non-keratinized
2. Stippling seen	Stippling not present
3. Pale pink in color	Comparatively red
4. It is firm and resilient	Loose and movable
5. Continuous with the marginal gingiva	Separated from attached gingiva by mucogingival junction.

Contd.

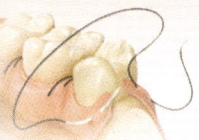

Contd.

Attached gingiva	Alveolar mucosa
6. Schiller's potassium iodide used to distinguish alveolar mucosa from attached gingiva.	Tension test is used to identify the mucogingival junction.

19. Manual and automated probing

Criteria	Manual probing	Automated probing
1. Probing force	Non-standardize	Constant and standardize
2. Applicability	Non-invasive and easy to use	Non-invasive, light weight and easy to use
3. Angulation	Subjective	Guidance system to ensure proper angulation
4. Readout	Manual	Direct electronic reading digital output
5. Tactile sensation	Full	Lacks
6. Reproducibility	Variable	Less variable
7. Cost-effectiveness	Cheapest	Very costly

20. Tooth and implant (Fig. 3.3)

Tooth	Implant
1. Periodontal ligament surrounds tooth root	No resilient connection between implants and supporting bone. Direct implant bone connection.
2. Tooth can intrude or drift in response to altered occlusal forces	Implant cannot change its position in any case.
3. Proprioceptive mechanism present in natural dentition	Lack of proprioception which reduces tactile sensitivity and reflex action.
4. Natural teeth continue to erupt during growth.	Implant cannot be placed in growing individuals.

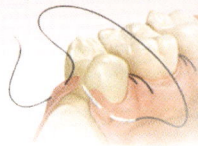

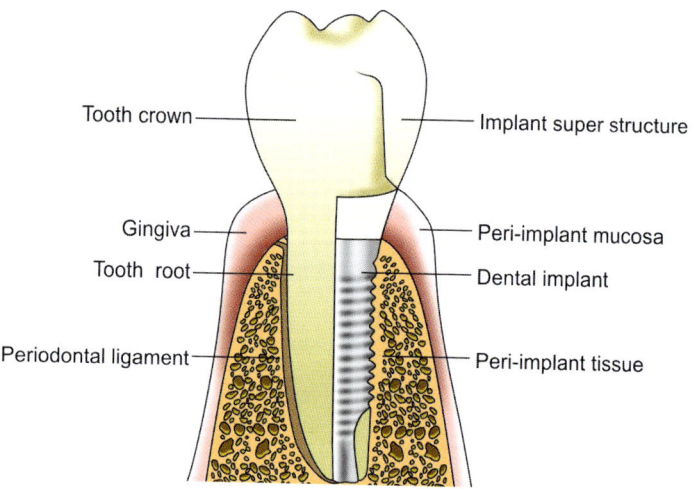

Tooth crown

Implant super structure

Gingiva

Peri-implant mucosa

Tooth root

Dental implant

Periodontal ligament

Peri-implant tissue

Fig. 3.3: Tooth *vs* implant

21. Gracey and universal curette

Gracey curette	Universal curette
1. Set of 14 (+4 modifications) curettes designed for specific areas and surfaces	One curette designed for all areas and surfaces
2. Only outer edge is cutting and hence work with either edges	Both the edges are cutting
3. Blade curves up and to the side; in two planes (Fig. 3.4A)	Blade curves only up; one plane only (Fig.3.4B)
4. Face of blade beveled at 60 degrees to the shank (Fig. 3.5A)	Face of the blade beveled at 90 degrees to shank (Fig. 3.5B)

A   B

Fig. 3.4: (A) Gracey curette, (B) Universal curette

A   B

Fig. 3.5: (A) Gracey curette, (B) Universal curette

22. Explorer and probe

Explorer	Probe
1. Used to check the smoothness of the root surface	Used to detect and measure the sulcus or pocket depth
2. It is used by tactile sensation to locate, detect the presence of subgingival calculus	It is used by introducing or "digging in" to the gingiva by certain amount of force.
3. The working end is thin, slender and sharp.	The working end is comparatively thick and blunt
4. Ex. #17, #23, Pigtail (Fig. 3.6)	Ex. Marquis color-coded probe, UNC 15 probe (Fig. 3.7)

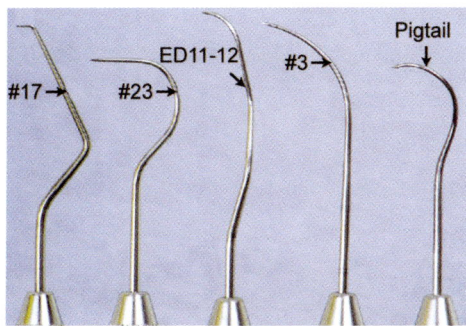

Fig. 3.6: Explorers

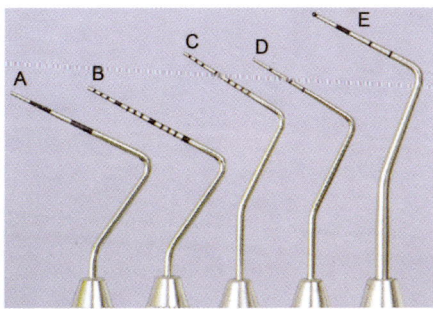

Fig. 3.7: Periodontal probes: (A) Marquis color-coded probe; (B) UNC 15 probe; (C) University of Michigan 'O' probe; (D) Michigan 'O' probe; (E) WHO probe

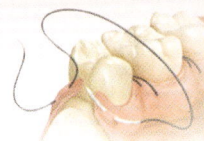

24. Primary and secondary trauma from occlusion (TFO)

Primary TFO	Secondary TFO
1. Tissue injury caused due to altered or increased occlusal forces	Tissue injury caused due to weakened periodontium (normal force), e.g. periodontitis
2. Tooth is tender on percussion, localized severe pain	Teeth may or may not be tender. Generalized dull pain may be present
3. Pocket is not present	Pockets may be present
4. Localized periodontal abscess may be present	Generalized swollen gingiva
5. Treated by occlusal adjustment	Treated by periodontal therapy
6. Bone loss is not evident	Bone loss present
7. Supracrestal fibers are unaffected	Supracrestal fibers are affected

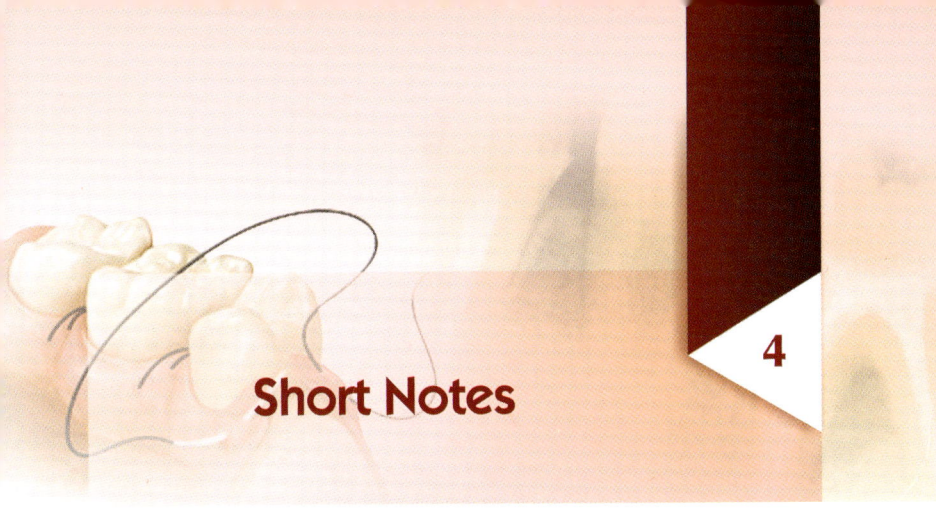

Short Notes

1. GINGIVAL SULCUS

The gingival sulcus is the shallow space between the free gingiva (unattached) and the tooth. It is 'V' shaped and barely permits the entrance of a periodontal probe. In clinically healthy gingiva, the sulcus depth varies from **2 to 3 mm.** (Penetration force 25 gm or 0.75N). The clinical determination of the depth of the gingival sulcus is an important diagnostic parameter. Under absolutely ideal conditions, (germfree animals) in absolute plaque control, gingival sulcus may be 0 or about 0. In fully erupted teeth, the gingival sulcus is lined with sulcular epithelium, the non-keratinized extension of the junctional epithelium (Fig. 4.1). Pathological deepening of sulcus is pocket. The gingival sulcus contains fluid that seeps into the sulcus from the basement membrane through the thin sulcular wall which is termed as gingival sulcular fluid.

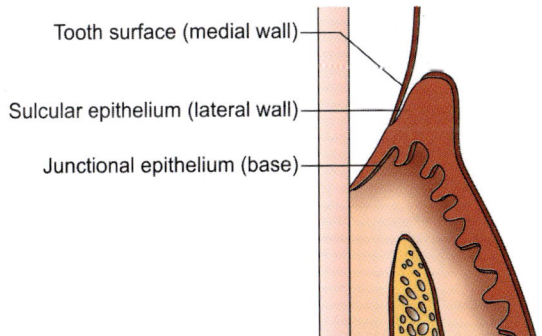

Tooth surface (medial wall)

Sulcular epithelium (lateral wall)

Junctional epithelium (base)

Fig. 4.1: Gingival sulcus

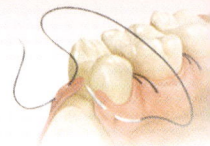

2. DEVELOPMENT OF THE GINGIVAL SULCUS

Once formation of enamel is complete, it is covered with reduced enamel epithelium (REE) which is attached to tooth by a basal lamina and hemidesmosomes. When the tooth ruptures the oral mucosa, the union of REE and the oral epithelium takes place; which is later called the junctional epithelium. After tooth eruption, this junctional epithelium condenses along the crown, and the ameloblasts, which form the inner layer of the REE, get converted into squamous epithelial cells. The transformation of the REE into junctional epithelium proceeds apically without interrupting the attachment to the tooth. Gingival sulcus forms at the time of tooth eruption. At this time, junctional epithelium and REE form a broad band attached to the tip of the tooth surface to the cementoenamel junction. As the tooth erupts only junctional epithelium persists forming a V-shaped crevice encircling the newly erupted crown.

3. ATTACHED GINGIVA

The part of gingiva which is continuous with the marginal gingiva is attached gingiva. It is firm, resilient and tightly bound to the underlying periosteum of the alveolar bone. The width of the attached gingiva on the facial aspect differs in different areas. The facial aspect of the attached gingiva extends to the relatively loose and movable alveolar mucosa from which it is demarcated by the mucogingival junction. The widest area found on the maxillary (3.5 to 4.5 mm) and mandibular incisors (3.5 to 3.9 mm), decreases toward canine region. The narrowest zone of gingiva is found in the region of the maxillary and mandibular first premolars (1.9 to 1.8 mm) and usually in connection with frenum and muscle attachment.

Width of the attached gingiva is an important clinical parameter. It is the distance between the mucogingival junction and external surface of the base of gingival sulcus or the pocket. It differs from the width of the keratinized gingiva because the keratinized gingiva also includes the marginal gingiva which is free or unattached.

The firmness and resiliency of attached gingiva may be because of the tight attachment of the connective tissue fibers to the cementum and bone. The gingiva is covered by keratinized or parakeratinized epithelium, the surface of which presents minute depressions and elevations, giving the surface an orange-peel appearance, known as stippling.

The width of attached gingiva increases with age and in supraerupted teeth. On the lingual aspect of the mandible, the attached gingiva terminates at the junction with the lingual alveolar mucosa. The palatal surface of the attached gingiva in the maxilla blends with the equally firm, resilient palatal mucosa.

4. COL AND ITS SIGNIFICANCE

The gingival tissue that extends interdentally forms gingival papillae. The valley-like depression that connects a facial and lingual papillae and conforms to the shape of interproximal contact is called as 'Col' (Fig. 4.2). At the eruption time and thereafter, col is covered by reduced enamel epithelium derived from approximating teeth which is gradually replaced by stratified squamous epithelium from adjacent interdental papillae.

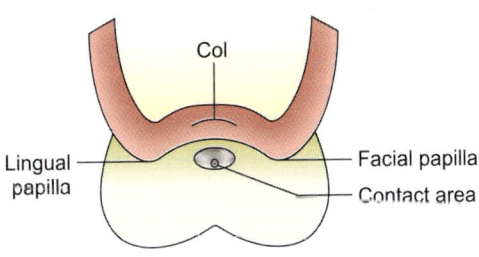

Fig. 4.2: Col

The interdental gingiva can be pyramidal or 'col' shaped. In pyramidal shape, the tip of papilla is immediately beneath the contact point. The shape of gingiva in the interdental space depends on the contact point between the two adjoining teeth and presence/absence of recession. The inflammatory process in gingivitis affects the sulcular and col epithelium along with

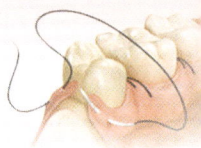

its underlying connective tissue. The products of the bacterial plaque located adjacent to or within the gingival sulcus or col first cause a disruption of the junctions and intercellular substances that hold the epithelial cells in these areas together. The loosening of the intercellular epithelial junctions provides larger pathways for the irritating plaque products to follow down into the connective tissues of the gingiva. The col is non-keratinized, hence the disease process progresses easily in the interdental gingiva.

5. GINGIVAL FIBERS

The connective tissue of the marginal gingiva is known as the lamina propria. The lamina propria of the marginal gingiva is densely collagenous, containing a prominent system of collagen fiber bundles called the gingival fibers. The functions of these fibers are:

1. To brace the marginal gingiva firmly against the tooth,
2. To provide rigidity necessary to withstand the forces of mastication without being deflected away from the tooth surface, and
3. To unite the free marginal gingiva with the cementum of the root and the adjacent attached gingiva.

The gingival fibers are arranged in three groups:

A. **Gingivodental group:** These are the fibers of the facial, lingual and interproximal surfaces. They are embedded in the cementum just beneath the base of the gingival sulcus. On the facial and lingual surfaces, they project from the cementum in a fan-like manner toward the crest and outer surface of marginal gingiva. They also extend externally to the periosteum and terminate in the attached gingiva or blend with the periosteum. Interproximally, extend towards the crest of the interdental gingiva (Fig. 4.3).

B. **Circular group:** These fibers encircle the tooth in the ring-like fashion through the connective tissue of marginal and interdental gingiva.

C. **Transseptal group:** These are located interproximally, extend between the cementum of approximating teeth into

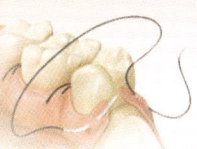

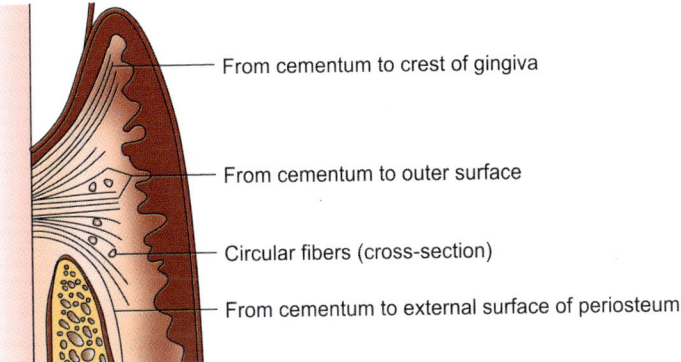

— From cementum to crest of gingiva

— From cementum to outer surface

— Circular fibers (cross-section)

— From cementum to external surface of periosteum

Fig. 4.3: Gingival fibers

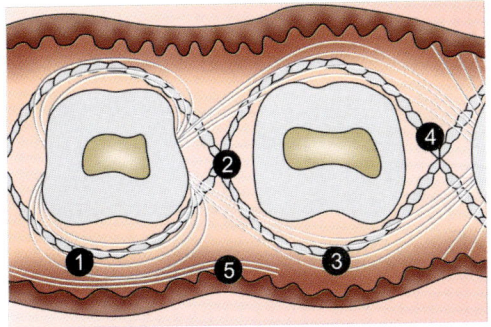

1. Semicircular fibers   2,4. Figure of 8 fibers
3. Transgingival fibers   5. Intragingival fibers

Fig. 4.4: Gingival fibers

which they are embedded. They lie in the area between the epithelium at the base of the gingival sulcus and the crest of the interdental bone. Transseptal fibers also classified with the principal fibers of the periodontal ligament.

Groups of semicircular and transgingival fibers have also been described (Fig. 4.4).

6. GINGIVAL PIGMENTATION

Melanin Pigmentation

Pigment containing cells, the melanocytes, are present in the basal layer of the gingival epithelium. "Melanin": non-hemoglobin derived brown pigment, is responsible for the

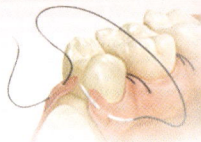

normal pigmentation of the skin, gingiva and remainder of the oral mucous membrane. It is present in all normal individuals and is absent or severely diminished in albinos. It is prominent in blacks (Fig. 4.5).

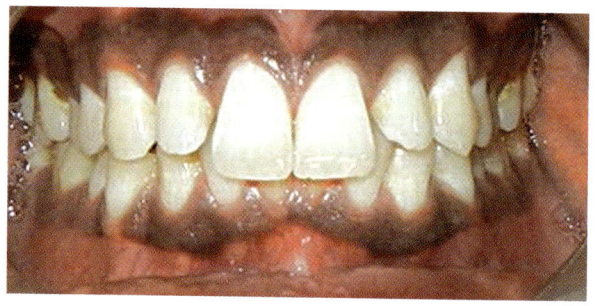

Fig. 4.5: Melanin pigmentation of the gingiva

Gingival pigmentation occurs as a diffuse, deep purplish discoloration or as irregularly shaped brown and light brown patches. It may appear in the gingiva as early as 3 hours after birth and often is the only evidence of pigmentation. Many systemic diseases may cause color changes in the oral mucosa including the gingiva.

In general, these abnormal pigmentations are nonspecific in nature. These may be endogenous or/and exogenous.

Endogenous Pigmentations

Endogenous oral pigmentations may be due to melanin, bilirubin, or iron. Addison's disease produces isolated patches of discoloration varying from bluish black to brown; Peutz-Jeghers syndrome also produces melanin pigmentation in the oral mucosa and lips.

Other systemic conditions producing pigmentation are hemochromatosis, diabetes, pregnancy, anemia, polycythemia and leukemia.

Pigmentation due to Exogenous Factors

Exogenous factors capable of producing color changes in the gingiva include atmospheric irritants such as coal, metal dust, coloring agents in food, tobacco, etc.

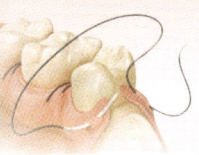

Metallic Pigmentation

Heavy metals (bismuth, arsenic, mercury, lead and silver) produce a black or bluish line in the gingiva which follows the contour of the margin. Lead results in a bluish red or deep blue linear pigmentation of the gingival margin (Burtonian line). Exposure to silver causes a violet marginal line. Localized bluish black areas of pigment are commonly due to amalgam implanted in the mucosa. Gingival pigmentation usually occurs in the areas of inflammation.

7. GINGIVAL STIPPLING AND ITS SIGNIFICANCE

The surface of the gingiva is characterized by an orange peel-like appearance called stippling. It may be fine or coarse and may vary in different individuals. It may also vary according to age and sex. It is absent in infancy, appears at about 5–6 years of age, increases until adulthood and frequently disappears after extraction/exfoliation of teeth or in old age.

Stippling is best viewed by drying the gingiva. The attached gingiva is stippled, the marginal gingiva is not. The central core of the interdental papilla is usually stippled. It is less prominent on lingual than on facial surfaces and may be absent in some persons. The pattern and extent of stippling varies from person to person and in different areas of the same mouth.

Stippling is because of alternate rounded protuberances and depressions in the gingival surface.

Stippling is a form of adaptive specialization or reinforcement for function. It is a feature of healthy gingiva and reduction or loss of stippling is a common sign of gingival disease. At the same time when the gingiva is restored to health following treatment, the stippling returns.

8. MICROSCOPIC PICTURE OF HEALTHY GINGIVA

Microscopically, gingiva consists of a central core of connective tissue covered by stratified squamous epithelium. The epithelium covering the marginal and attached gingivae is either parakeratinized or keratinized while the sulcular and junctional epithelia are non-keratinized.

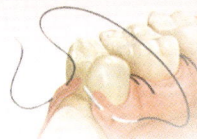

The oral epithelium has four layers. The principal cells of oral epithelium are **'Keratinocytes'**. The first cell layer lying on the basement membrane composed of cuboidal cells (stratum basale). The second layer the stratum spinosum composed of polygonal cells, (prickle cell layer). The third layer of flattened cells, the stratum granulosum, containing lamellated granules. These granules are modified lysosomes and are called Odland bodies or keratinosomes. The most superficial layer, the stratum corneum, consists of flat cells. The epithelial cells are joined together by structures known as desmosomes (Fig. 4.6).

Turnover rate of palate, tongue and cheek is 5 to 6 days, while that of gingiva is 10 to 12 days, in experimental animals.

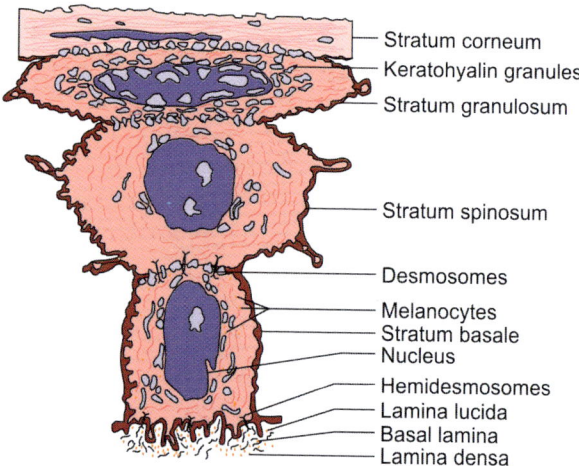

Stratum corneum
Keratohyalin granules
Stratum granulosum

Stratum spinosum

Desmosomes
Melanocytes
Stratum basale
Nucleus
Hemidesmosomes
Lamina lucida
Basal lamina
Lamina densa

Fig. 4.6: Microscopic structure of gingival epithelium

Nonkeratinocytes

1. **Langerhans cells:** These are dendritic cells present at all suprabasal levels among the keratinocytes. They have antigenic property, so are considered as macrophages. These are absent in the junctional epithelium.

2. **Merkel cells:** These are terminals of nerve fibers connected to adjacent cells by desmosomes. They are located in the deeper layers of epithelium and are tactile perception cells.

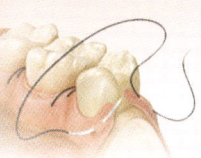

3. **Melanocytes:** These are dendritic cells located in the basal and spinous layers of gingival epithelium. They synthesize melanin in organelles called premelanosomes. Melanin granules phagocytozed by other cells are called as melanophages or melanophores.

The basement membrane or basal lamina is the junction between epithelium and the connective tissue. It is 300–400 Å thick and composed of lamina densa (adjacent to the connective tissue) and lamina lucida (adjacent to the epithelium). Basal lamina is permeable to fluids.

The connective tissue of the gingiva is known as lamina propria which is divided into two layers: (i) The papillary layer—adjacent to the epithelium, and (ii) The reticular layer—towards the periosteum of the alveolar bone. It consists of collagen fibers, intercellular ground substance, cells, blood vessels, and nerves.

The connective tissue also contains inflammatory cells, such as plasma cells, mast cells and lymphocytes.

9. JUNCTIONAL EPITHELIUM

The junctional epithelium is formed by the union or fusion of the oral epithelium and the reduced enamel epithelium during tooth eruption. It is a collar-like band of stratified squamous non-keratinizing epithelium. The junctional epithelium is attached to the tooth surface (epithelial attachment) by internal basal lamina and to the gingival connective tissue by an external basal lamina. The internal basal lamina consists of lamina densa (adjacent to the enamel) and of lamina lucida to which hemidesmosomes are attached. Hemidesmosomes have a decisive role in the firm attachment of the cells to the internal basal lamina on the tooth surface.

The thickness of the junctional epithelium ranges from 3 to 4 layers in early life and increases to 10 to 20 layers with age. The length of the junctional epithelium ranges from 0.25 to 1.35 mm. It is continually self-renewing structure with mitotic activity occurring in all cell layers. Hence, it is completely restored after pocket therapy or surgery.

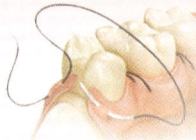

The attachment of the junctional epithelium to the tooth surface is reinforced by the gingival fibers, for this reason, the junctional epithelium and gingival fibers are considered as a functional unit, the **dentogingival unit**. Hence, the junctional epithelium exhibits several structural and functional features such as:

1. Forming an epithelial barrier against bacteria
2. Allows access of gingival fluid, inflammatory cells hence host defense
3. Rapid turnover of epithelial cells and rapid repair.

10. CLINICAL FEATURES OF HEALTHY GINGIVA (Fig. 4.7)

These are as follows:

1. **Color:** The color of the marginal and attached gingiva is described as coral pink, and is produced by the vascular supply, the thickness and keratinization of the epithelium. The attached gingiva is demarcated from the adjacent alveolar mucosa on buccal aspect by a clearly defined mucogingival line. The alveolar mucosa is red, smooth, shiny and thin.

   The gingiva may be pigmented, if melanin producing cells are present in basal cell layer of the epithelium.

2. **Contour or shape:** The marginal gingiva encircles the teeth in collar-like fashion, and follows scalloped outline on the facial and lingual surfaces. The interdental gingiva or papilla is pyramidal in the anterior region whereas the papilla is more flattened in the buccolingual direction in the posterior region.

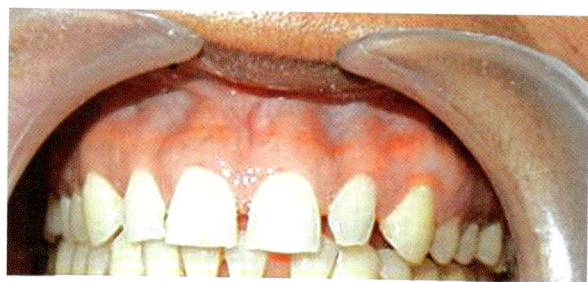

Fig. 4.7: Clinical picture of healthy gingiva

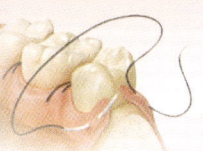

3. **Consistency:** The consistency of the gingiva is resilient and firm and tightly bound to the underlying bone.

4. **Size:** The size of the gingiva corresponds to the sum total of the bulk of cellular and intercellular elements and their vascular supply.

5. **Surface texture:** Surface texture is determined by presence of stippling. The attached gingiva is stippled and not the marginal gingiva. The central portion of the interdental papilla is usually stippled. The appearance is that of an orange peel. It varies from person to person with pattern and extent. It is less prominent on lingual than facial surfaces and may be absent in some individuals. It is a significant clinical characteristic of normal gingiva.

6. **Position:** It is the level at which the gingival margin is attached to the tooth surface. Usually, it is correlated to cementoenamel junction.

   In short, clinical features of healthy gingiva are c^3s^2p.

11. FUNCTIONS OF THE PERIODONTAL LIGAMENT

The functions of the periodontal ligament (PDL) are:

Physical: The physical functions of the periodontal ligament are: (a) Transmission of occlusal forces to the bone, (b) attachment of the teeth to the bone, (c) maintenance of the gingival tissues in their proper relationship to the teeth, (d) resistance to the impact of occlusal forces, (e) provisions of a "soft tissue casing" to protect the vessels and nerves from injury.

Formative: PDL cells take part in formation, resorption of cementum and bone and in the repair of injuries.

Remodeling: Old cells and fibers are broken down and replaced by new ones. Mitotic activity is observed in fibroblasts and endothelial cells. (Fibroblasts form collagen fibers, osteoblasts, cementoblasts.)

Thus rate of formation and differentiation of fibroblasts affects the rate of formation of collagen, cementum and bone.

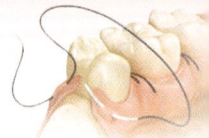

Nutritional: The periodontal ligament supplies nutrients to the cementum, bone, and gingiva, by way of blood vessels and provides lymphatic drainage.

Sensory: Nerve bundles pass into the PDL from periapical area and through channels from the alveolar bone that follows the course of blood vessels. The innervation of the periodontal ligament provides proprioceptive and tactile sensitivity by trigeminal pathways, which detects and localizes external forces acting upon the individual tooth/teeth.

12. RESISTANCE TO THE IMPACT OF OCCLUSAL FORCES (SHOCK–ABSORPTION)

Two theories have been considered:
1. The tensional theory
2. The viscoelastic system theory

1. The Tensional Theory

According to this theory, the principal fibers of the periodontal ligament are responsible in supporting the tooth and transmitting forces to the bone. When force is applied to the tooth, the principal fibers first unfold and straighten and then transmit forces to the alveolar bone, causing an elastic deformation of the bony socket. Finally when the alveolar bone has reached its limit, the load is transmitted to the basal bone.

2. The Viscoelastic Theory

According to this theory, the displacement of the tooth is largely controlled by fluid movements, with fibers having only a secondary role. When forces are transmitted to the tooth, the extracellular fluid passes from the periodontal ligament into the marrow spaces of bone through foramina in the cortical layer, which are more abundant in the cervical and middle third than the middle and apical thirds.

After the depletion of tissue fluids, the fiber bundles tighten. This leads to blood vessel stenosis, arterial back—pressure which causes ballooning of the vessels and passage of blood ultrafiltrates into the tissues, thereby replenishing the tissue fluids.

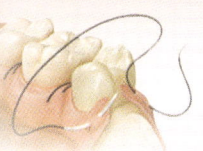

Transmission of occlusal forces to the bone: When an axial force is applied to a tooth, there is a tendency towards displacement of the root into the alveolus. The oblique fibers alter their wavy pattern, get straighten and sustain the major part of the axial force.

When a horizontal or tipping force is applied, there are two phases of tooth movement. The first is within the confines of the periodontal ligament and the bony plates. Secondly, the tooth rotates about an axis.

The apical portion of the root moves in a direction opposite to the coronal portion. In areas of tension, the principal fiber bundles are taut rather than wavy. In areas of pressure, the fibers are compressed.

13. PRINCIPAL FIBERS OF THE PERIODONTAL LIGAMENT

The periodontal ligament contains collagen fibers, which are inserted on one side in cementum and on the other side in alveolar bone. These fibers are arranged into groups called principal fiber bundles, and follow a wavy course when viewed in longitudinal section. The fibers that are inserted into cementum and bone are termed 'Sharpey's fibers', the terminal portions of the principal fibers.

The principal fibers are arranged in the following groups (Fig. 4.8):

1. **Transseptal group:** Interproximal fibers extend over the alveolar crest and are embedded in the cementum of adjacent teeth.

2. **Alveolar crest group:** These fibers extend obliquely from the cementum just beneath the junctional epithelium to the alveolar crest. They help in retaining the tooth in the socket.

3. **Horizontal group:** These fibers extend at right angles to the long-axis of the tooth from cementum to the alveolar bone.

4. **Oblique group:** The largest group extends from cementum in a coronal direction obliquely to the bone. These fibers bear most of the vertical masticatory forces.

5. **Apical group:** They radiate from cementum to the bone at the apical region of the socket.

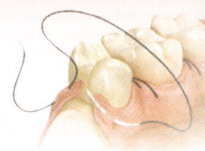

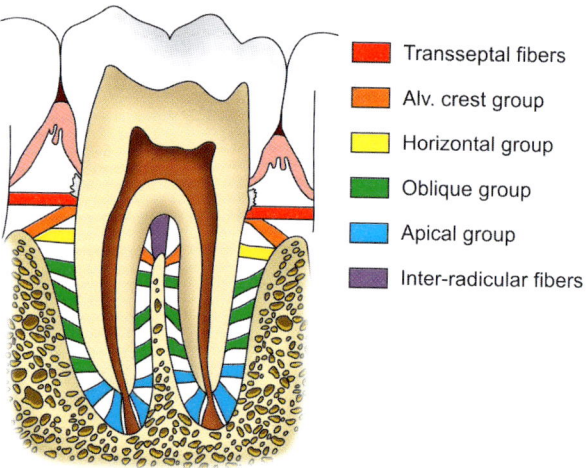

Fig. 4.8: Principal fibers of periodontal ligament

6. **Inter-radicular group:** This group courses from cementum to bone in the furcation of multi-rooted teeth.

Apart from the principal fibers, oxytalan, elunine and elastic fibers are also present.

14. INTERMEDIATE PLEXUS

The principal fiber bundles consist of individual fibers that form a continuous anastomosing network between tooth and bone. It has been suggested that instead of using continuous, the individual fibers consist of two separate parts spliced together midway between cementum and bone in a zone called the intermediate plexus.

The concept of an intermediate plexus in human arose from the study of the erupting tooth and from the observation of an apparent mingling of the alveolar and cemental fibers near the center of the ligament, permitted the rearrangement of fibers during eruptive and migratory tooth movements. There are doubts regarding the existence of such plexus, and if at all it exists, it disappears after the tooth come in contact with its antagonists.

The existence of such a plexus has not been confirmed by radiographic data and some consider it as a microscopic artifact.

15. THE CEMENTOENAMEL JUNCTION

The cementum at cementoenamel junction is of particular clinical importance in root scaling and root planing procedures. Three types of relationships involving the cementum may exist at cementoenamel junction (Fig. 4.9). In about 60–65% of cases cementum overlaps the enamel while in 30% there is an edge butt joint and in 5 to 10% cases, cementum and enamel fail to meet. Therefore, in last, i.e. 5 to 10% cases, gingival recession may be present along with root sensitivity due to exposed dentin.

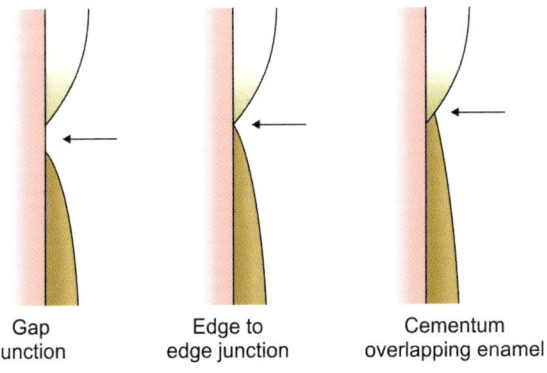

| Gap junction | Edge to edge junction | Cementum overlapping enamel |

Fig. 4.9: Cementoenamel junctions

16. CEMENTUM AND ITS BIOLOGIC IMPORTANCE

Cementum is calcified tissue that covers the root of the tooth and provides a means of attachment for the periodontal ligament fibers to the tooth. Cementum is continuously formed on the root surfaces, which is necessary for the maintenance of healthy periodontium. Cementum formation and deposition is most rapid in the apical regions, where it compensates for tooth attrition. This function of the cementum is useful for the maintenance of vertical dimension of occlusion throughout life.

Hypercementosis: It refers to a prominent thickening of cementum. It generally results from excessive tension from orthodontic appliances or from occlusal forces. In teeth without antagonist, hypercementosis occurs as an effort to keep pace with excessive tooth eruption. In teeth, subject to low grade

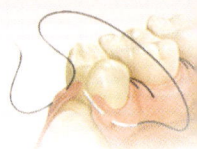

periapical irritation arising from pulp disease, it is considered to be the compensation for the destroyed fibrous attachment to the tooth. The cementum is deposited adjacent to the inflamed periapical tissue.

Cementum resorption: The cementum of erupted and unerupted teeth is subject to resorption. It may be due to local and systemic conditions. Local causes are trauma from occlusion, orthodontic movement, pressure from malaligned erupting teeth, cysts and tumors, teeth without functional antagonists, replanted or transplanted teeth, periapical and periodontal disease. Systemic causes are—calcium deficiency, hypothyroidism and Paget's disease.

Role of cementum: An unclacified layer of precementum, part of the process of continuous cementum deposition, was considered to be the natural barrier to excessive apical migration of junctioinal epithelium.

Impaired cementum formation (cementopathy) was thought to be a cause of pathologic periodontal pocket formation, because it reduced the restrain on epithelium migration. Cementum resorption and repair is also important during the orthodontic therapy.

Due to periodontal disease, the cementum gets diseased and allows the toxins, enzymes liberated by the micro-organism to get deposited in cemental pores. After treatment, it has a capacity to get reformed for better attachment of gingival and periodontal ligament fibers, hence minimizing the pocket depth and improving the attachment to the tooth. The importance of cementum, in forensic odontology, for estimation of age of the individual is considered.

17. ANKYLOSIS

The fusion of cementum and alveolar bone with obliteration of periodontal ligament represents a form of abnormal repair and occurs in teeth with cemental resorption. When titanium implants are placed in the jaw, healing results in formation of bone in direct apposition to the implant without any intervening tissue. In this kind of ankylosis, because resorption of the

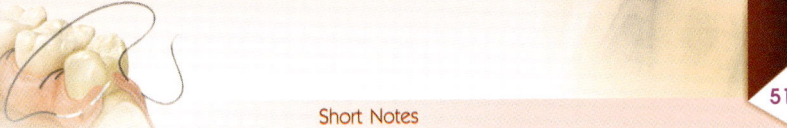
metallic implant cannot occur, the implant remains indefinitely "ankylosed" to the bone. Also, because apical proliferation of the epithelium along the root, a key element of pocket formation is not possible owing to ankylosis, a true periodontal pocket will not be formed.

18. FUNCTIONS OF CEMENTUM

1. Acellular extrinsic fiber cementum anchors the tooth via principal fibers to alveolar bone.
2. Cellular intrinsic fiber cementum participates in repair process unrelated to external root resorption lacunae, intra-alveolar root fracture and closure of apical foramina following apisectomy.
3. Cellular intrinsic fiber cementum also regulates homeostasis, i.e. cementocytes being engaged in cementolysis.

19. FENESTRATIONS AND DEHISCENCES

These are the defects in the alveolar process. The alveolar **Fenestration** is a circumscribed window in the cortical plate over the root and does not communicate with the crestal margin or it is an isolated area or areas where the root is denuded of bone and the root surface is covered only by periosteum and overlying gingiva. In this case, marginal bone is intact (Fig. 4.10).

Dehiscence: It is a dipping of the crestal bone margin exposing the root surface or when the denuded areas extend through

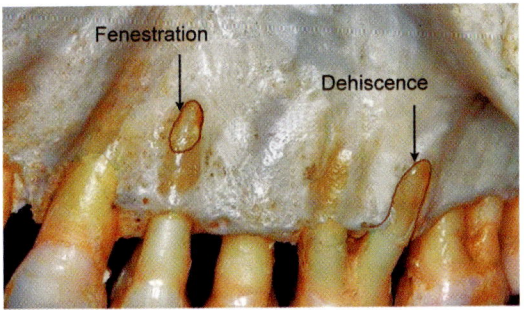

Fig. 4.10: Fenestration and dehiscence

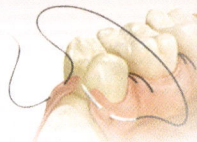

the marginal bone exposing complete root. Such defects occur on approximately 20% of the teeth. They occur more often on the facial bone than on the lingual and are commonly on anterior teeth than posterior teeth, and are usually bilateral. The etiology is not known, but trauma from occlusion may be suspected. The predisposing factors are prominent root contours, malposition of teeth, thin bony plates, labial protrusion of root, etc.

These defects are important to a periodontist because they may complicate the outcome of periodontal surgery.

20. PERIOSTEUM AND ENDOSTEUM

Tissue covering the outer surface of the bone is periosteum; while the tissue lining the internal bony cavities is called endosteum. Endosteum is single layer of osteoblasts and small amount of connective tissue. Both periosteum and endosteum have osteogenic potential.

There are two layers of periosteum—inner layer rich in osteoblasts surrounded by osteoprogenitor cells and outer layer rich in blood vessels, nerves and fibers.

Periosteum is tightly adhered to underlying bone through the bundles of periosteal collagen fibers; penetrating into it. It modulates the balance between bone formation and resorption. Osteogenic potential of periosteum is important in periodontal plastic surgical procedures, regenerative periodontics and tissue engineering.

21. AGING AND THE PERIODONTIUM

Aging is a slowing down of natural function due to changes which may be intrinsic and chronologically related, or may be extrinsic and attributable to the environment. The changes affect following tissues:

Vasculature: Arteriosclerosis is a frequent finding in aging; it may be seen in the vessels of alveolar bone and periodontal ligament. The blood supply is reduced with fragility of capillaries resulting in reduced oxygen consumption.

Gingiva and mucosa: Diminished keratinization with reduced stippling and increased width of attached gingiva. Decreased

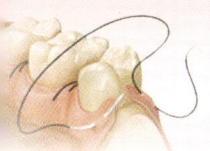

connective tissue cellularity with greater amount of intercellular substances is noted. The oxygen consumption rate is reduced. The overall oral epithelium is thin. There is increased keratinization of lip and cheek mucosa, atrophy of the connective tissue with loss of elasticity, a decrease in the number of protein bound hexoses and mucoproteins and an increase in the number of mast cells.

Periodontal ligament: Aging results in greater number of elastic fibers, decrease in vascularity, altered cell permeability and increased calcium content, mitotic activity and the number of collagen fibers. The reduction of width of periodontal ligament is evident.

A decrease in width due to lower functional demands owing to the decrease in strength of masticatory musculature or encroachment on periodontal ligament due to continuous deposition of bone and cementum. Sometimes an increase in width may be due to availability of fewer teeth to support the entire functional load.

Alveolar bone and cementum: In bone, there is osteoporosis, decreased vascularity and reduction in metabolic rate and healing capacity. Bone resorption activity may be increased or decreased. The rate of bone formation is decreased.

There is greater irregularity in the surfaces of bone and cementum with continuous increase in the amount of cementum.

Tooth–periodontium relationships: Occlusal wear reduces cusp height and inclination of teeth with a resultant increase in the food table area and loss of sluiceways. The degree of attrition is more likely to be the result of unreplaced missing teeth, loose teeth, poorly fitting dentures, or an unwillingness to wear dentures.

Other Changes

1. Alteration in plaque and immune response
2. Xerostomia
3. Reparative, transparent and sclerotic dentin
4. Pulp reduces in size.

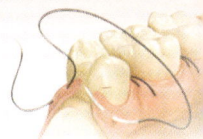

22. CLASSIFICATION OF THE GINGIVAL DISEASES

I. Dental Plaque-induced Gingival Lesions

a. Gingivitis associated with plaque only:
  i. Marginal gingivitis,
  ii. Papillary gingivitis,
  iii. Diffuse gingivitis.
  (It can be either localized or generalized.)
b. Gingival diseases modified by systemic factors
  i. Associated with endocrine system
    1. Hormonal
    2. Diabetics
  ii. Associated with blood dyscrasias, e.g. leukemia
c. Gingival diseases modified by medications, e.g. drug-induced gingival enlargement
d. Gingival diseases modified by malnutrition, e.g. scurvy (vitamin C defficiency)

II. Non-plaque-induced Gingival Lesions

a. Gingival diseases of specific bacterial origin, e.g. *Neisseria gonorrhoeae*
b. Gingival diseases of viral origin, e.g. herpes virus infection.
c. Gingival infections of fungal origin, e.g. candidal infection.
d. Gingival lesions of genetic origin, e.g. hereditary gingival fibromatosis.
e. Gingival manifestation of systemic conditions.
  i. Mucocutaneous lesions, e.g. lichen planus.
  ii. Allergic reactions to the dental restorative materials, dentifrices or others
f. Traumatic lesions (physical, chemical or thermal injury)
g. Foreign body reactions.
h. Non-specific

23. CLASSIFICATION OF PERIODONTITIS

Diseases

  I. Chronic periodontitis—localized and generalized
  II. Aggressive periodontitis—localized and generalized

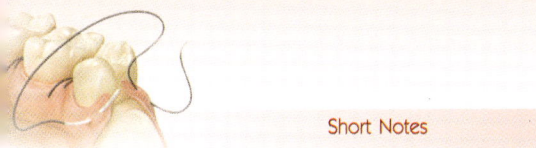

III. Refractory periodontitis
IV. Periodontitis as a manifestation of systemic diseases:
    a. Hematologic disorders, e.g. leukemias
    b. Genetic disorders, e.g. Down's syndrome
    c. Not otherwise specified

Conditions

   I. Necrotizing periodontal disease—necrotizing ulcerative periodontitis.
  II. Abscesses of the periodontium—periodontal abscess, pericoronal abscess.
 III. Periodontitis associate with endodontic lesions:
    – Primary perio—secondary endo lesion
    – Primary endo—secondary perio lesion
    – Combined lesion.
 IV. Developmental or acquired deformities or conditions:
    – Localized tooth related factors
    – Mucogingival deformities and conditions around teeth.
    – Mucogingival deformities and conditions on edentulous ridges
    – Occlusal trauma.

24. PREVALENCE OF GINGIVAL AND PERIODONTAL DISEASE

Various epidemiological studies worldwide and in India suggest higher prevalence of gingival and periodontal disease. Compared to western countries, the severity of periodontal disease is higher in Asian countries.

This may be attributed to:
– Low socioeconomic status
– Lack of awareness.
– Psychological and cultural barrier.
– Lack of sufficient and professional dental care.

Sex: In general, gingival and periodontal disease is distributed equally in males and females. Females are usually affected

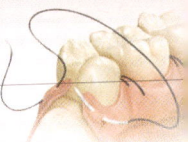

because of hormonal changes while males predispose to periodontal disease due to various tobacco habits and stress.

Age: Although periodontal disease is more observed in adults above 40 years of age, it can be seen at all ages except in children with deciduous dentition. Prevalence is around 1 to 2%.

Diet: Periodontal disease is more evident among consumers of soft and sticky food and malnourished individuals.

Socioeconomic status: Lower income group have higher rate of periodontal disease than higher income group. This is directly related to unaffordability of low socioeconomic group for costly dental services.

Other factors: Dental caries, malocclusion, tobacco habits, education, other systemic diseases and conditions, such as diabetes and HIV infection, are the contributing factors in the wide-spread prevalence of periodontal disease.

25. GINGIVAL FLUID/GINGIVAL CREVICULAR FLUID (GCF)

The gingival sulcus contains a fluid that seeps into the sulcus from the gingival connective tissue through the thin sulcular wall. The gingival fluid plays a protective role. Several mechanisms have been suggested:

1. Cleansing action, based on the flushing out of bacteria and particulate matter.
2. Antibacterial properties, based on its content of viable leukocytes that can engulf and destroy bacteria.
3. Antibodies against plaque bacteria.
4. Adhesive properties, based on the presence of sticky plasma proteins, which may improve adhesions of junctional epithelium to the tooth.

Female sex hormones increase the gingival fluid flow:

Collection of GCF: There are different methods of collection:

1. Absorbing paper strips,
2. Microcapillary pipets, and
3. Gingival washing.

The amount of fluid collected on a paper strip can be evaluated in a variety of ways: On a blotter (perio paper), employing an electronic transducer (Periotron). The amount

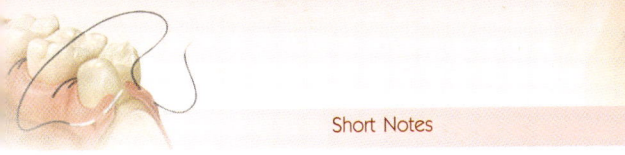

of gingival fluid is greater when inflammation is present, sometimes proportional to its severity. Therefore, it is considered as inflammatory exudate.

Clinical significance: Analysis of GCF constitutes in health and disease is helpful in detecting and diagnosing active disease or to predict patients at risk. GCF is increased by:

1. Mastication of coarse foods.
2. Tooth brushing and gingival massage.
3. Ovulation and hormonal contraceptives.
4. Smoking
5. Circadian periodicity, i.e. 6 AM to 10 PM
6. Periodontal therapy.

Drugs, like tetracycline and metronidazole, are excreted in the GCF and can be used advantageously in periodontal therapy.

Thus the composition of GCF provides knowledge that it could be one of the noninvasive procedures for the detection and treatment of periodontal diseases.

26. ROLE OF SALIVA IN ORAL HEALTH

Saliva is protective in nature as it maintains the oral tissues in physiologic state. Following components and physical properties are responsible for the protective nature of saliva:

1. Glycoproteins and mucoids offer coating similar to gastric mucin and hence physically protect the oral structures and also act as a lubricant; thereby preventing tooth desiccation.
2. Their physical flow causes clearance of debris and bacteria thereby enhancing the mechanical cleansing.
3. Salivary bicarbonates and phosphates buffer acids produced by bacteria, hence act as an antacid.
4. Minerals present in saliva help in both maturation and remineralization thereby maintaining the tooth integrity.
5. IgA present in saliva controls bacterial colonization.
6. Lysozyme in saliva breaks the bacterial cell wall leading to bactericidal effect.

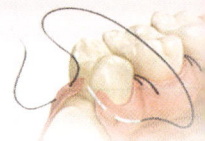

7. Salivary lactoperoxidase causes oxidation of susceptible bacteria.

27. STAGES OF GINGIVITIS

There are mainly three stages of gingivitis before extending into the alveolar bone or PDL.

Stage I gingivitis/subclinical gingivitis/initial lesion: Dilated capillaries and increased blood flow in response to microbial activation of local leukocytes is evident. At the same time perivascular loss of collagen is also noted.

Clinical changes are not apparent except increase in the GCF flow. If this lesion does not resolve on its own within 5 days, it leads to stage II.

Stage II gingivitis/early gingivitis/early lesion: Macrophages and lymphocytes appear at the site along with the infiltration of leukocytes in the connective tissue (mainly lymphocytes with majority T cells). Junctional epithelium starts to develop rete pegs. Collagen loss takes place around inflammatory infiltrate. Neutrophils migrate through epithelium to gingival sulcus. Various stages of phagocytosis are observed.

Clinically, erythematous changes appear in gingiva with bleeding on probing. This stage may last for 4 to 7 days or even for weeks together.

Stage III gingivitis/chronic gingivitis/established lesion: Predominant and primary histologic characteristic of this stage is the presence of plasma cells and B lymphocytes (especially IgG_1 and IgG_3). Engorged blood vessels with impaired venous return are noted. Widened intercellular spaces are seen in junctional epithelium filled with cellular debris and lysosomes. Protruding rete pegs of junctional epithelium with loss of basal lamina in some areas also observed along with the continued loss of collagen around infiltrate.

Clinically, gingiva gets bluish hue due to venous stenosis and breakdown of extravasated hemoglobin in connective tissue. Gingival edema and reduced stippling may be noted at this stage (occurs within 2 to 3 weeks).

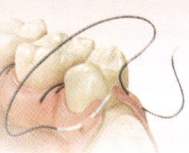

In some individuals, stage III of gingivitis may remain stable for months together without progressing further. However, it may become more active and leads to progressively destructive lesion.

Elimination of local irritants can reverse the lesion back to normal in any of the above stages. But, if not, inflammation can extend to alveolar bone and PDL causing periodontal destruction.

28. CLINICAL FEATURES OF GINGIVITIS

It may be characterized by the presence of any of the following clinical signs:

Color change: Normal gingival color is coral pink and is produced by the tissue vascularity and modified by overlying epithelial layers. Therefore, gingiva appears red in acute exacerbation, pale in fibrosis and red to bluish red in chronic gingivitis. Color changes start from interdental papilla, gingival margin and spread to attached gingiva.

Change in gingival consistency: Consistency of normal gingiva is firm and resilient. In chronic gingivitis, both destructive (edematous) and reparative (fibrotic) changes coexist, and the consistency of gingiva is determined by their relative predominance. Therefore, consistency differs from soft and edematous to firm and leathery in diseased condition.

Changes in surface texture of the gingiva: The surface of normal gingiva usually exhibits stippling, which is restricted to attached gingiva and extends to a variable degree into the interdental papilla. In chronic inflammation, gingival surface is either smooth and shiny or firm and nodular, depending on whether the dominant changes are exudative or fibrotic. The stippling may get reduced or lost.

Change in position of gingiva: Position of the gingiva is level of marginal gingiva with respect to cementoenamel junction (CEJ). In disease condition, it can shift either coronal (gingival enlargement) or apical (gingival recession) to CEJ.

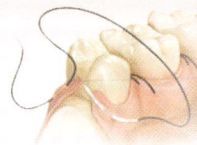

Change in contour: In normal condition, marginal gingiva is scalloped. In gingivitis, the change in contour may be in form of enlargement, Stillman's clefts or McCall festoons.

1. **Stillman's cleft:** It is a specific type of gingival recession consisting of a narrow, triangular-shaped gingival recession (Fig. 4.11).

2. **McCall festoons:** It is a rolled thickened band of gingiva usually seen adjacent to cuspids when recession approaches to mucogingival junction. Initially, Stillman's cleft and McCall festoons were attributed to traumatic occlusion (Fig. 4.12).

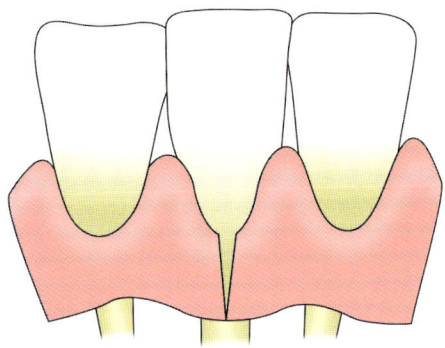

Fig. 4.11: Stillman's cleft

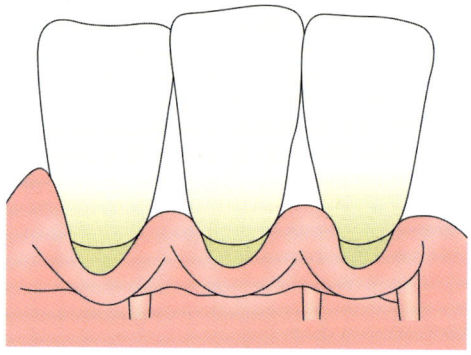

Fig. 4.12: McCall festoon

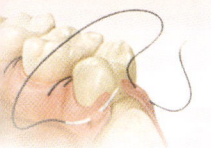

Bleeding on probing (BOP) (Fig. 4.13): Gingival bleeding can be easily detected clinically. Therefore, it is of value in early diagnosis and prevention of more advanced gingivitis. BOP appears earlier than a change in colour or other visual sings of inflammation. It indicates inflammatory lesion both in epithelium and connective tissue.

Above changes are seen along with presence of calculus or plaque, without radiographic evidence of crestal bone loss.

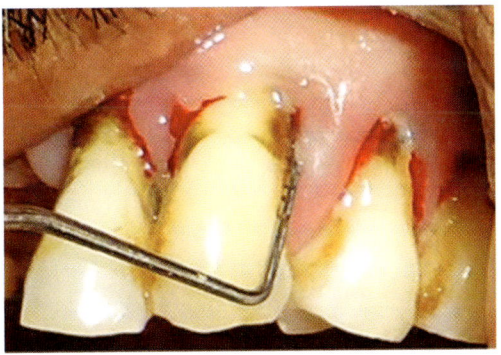

Fig. 4.13: Bleeding on probing

29. STILLMAN'S CLEFTS AND McCALL FESTOONS

Stillman's clefts are apostrophe-shaped indentation/narrow slits extending from and into the gingival margin in an apical direction for varying distance (Fig. 4.11). The clefts generally occur on the facial surface. One or two may be present in relation to a single tooth. At times, the clefts are linear and diagnosed on probing the gingival margin. The etiology of the clefts may be considered to be the result of occlusal trauma. They are also thought to be pathological pockets in which the ulcerative process has extended to the facial surface of the gingiva. The clefts may repair spontaneously or persist as surface lesions of deep periodontal pockets that penetrate into the supporting tissues.

The clefts are simple clefts with cleavage in a single direction, and compound clefts, wherein cleavage occurs in more than one direction. The clefts also can be true or pseudo. The clefts

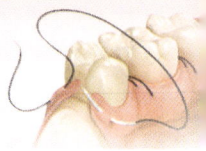

vary in length from as slight break in the gingival margin to a depth of 5 to 6 mm or more.

McCall festoons are life-saver shaped enlargements of the marginal gingiva (Fig. 4.12). The appearance of the marginal gingiva is rolled. McCall festoons are commonly seen in the canine and premolar areas on the facial surface. The etiology of festoons is considered to be the occlusal trauma.

30. GINGIVAL BLEEDING

Bleeding from gingival sulcus is the earliest sign and symptom of gingival inflammation. Bleeding on probing is clinically easily detectable and, therefore, of great value for the early diagnosis and, prevention, of more advanced gingivitis. It has been shown that bleeding on probing appears earlier than change in color or other visual signs of inflammation. Gingival bleeding is more objective sign, requiring less subjective estimation by the examiner. Gingival bleeding varies in severity, duration and the ease with which it is provoked.

Abnormal gingival bleeding is due to dilation and engorgement of the capillaries and thinning or ulceration of the sulcular epithelium. It can be acute, chronic or associated with systemic diseases.

Gingival bleeding caused due to local factors.

A. **Acute gingival bleeding:** It is caused by injury or occurs spontaneously in gingival disease. Laceration of the gingiva by tooth brush bristle or by sharp pieces of hard food causes gingival bleeding even in absence of disease. Gingival burns from hot foods or chemicals increase the ease of gingival bleeding.

Spontaneous bleeding occurs in ANUG. This may be because of the exposure of the blood vessels due to ulceration and necrosis.

B. **Chronic and recurrent bleeding:** The common cause of abnormal gingival bleeding is chronic inflammation. The bleeding is provoked by mechanical trauma, such as that from tooth brushing, tooth picks, or food impaction. Sites that bleed on probing have greater areas of inflamed cell

rich, collagen poor connective tissue. The severity of bleeding and the ease with which it is provoked depend on the intensity of the inflammation.

After the vessels rupture, a complex of mechanisms induces hemostasis. Bleeding recurs when tissue area is irritated.

In cases of moderate or advanced periodontitis, presence of bleeding on probing is considered a sign of active tissue destruction.

C. **Gingival bleeding associated with systemic disturbances:** There are certain systemic disorders in which gingival bleeding, occurs spontaneously and in such cases the control becomes difficult. The hemorrhagic tendency may be due to failure of one or more of the hemostatic mechanisms, such as vascular abnormalities, vitamin C and K deficiency, coagulation defects, like hemophilia, leukemia, etc. Bleeding may follow the administration of excessive amounts of drugs, such as salicylates, dicumurol or heparin. Excessive gingival bleeding may also be encountered during menstrual period and other related hormonal imbalance conditions.

31. CLASSIFICATION OF GINGIVAL ENLARGEMENT

I. Inflammatory enlargement
   - Chronic
   - Acute

II. Gingival hyperplasia (fibrotic enlargement)
   - Drug-induced gingival enlargement
   - Idiopathic

III. Combined gingival enlargement (inflammatory as well as fibrotic)

IV. Enlargement associated with systemic conditions or diseases.
   - Conditioned enlargement, e.g. puberty, pregnancy, scurvy, plasma cell gingivitis, nonspecific
   - Systemic diseases causing gingival enlargement, e.g. leukemia, granulomatous diseases.

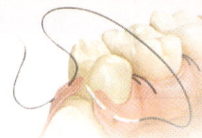

V. Neoplastic enlargement (gingival tumors)
- Benign
- Malignant

VI. False enlargement

Depending upon the distribution and involvement, gingival enlargement can be localized or generelized. It can also be marginal, papillary, diffuse or descrete.

Gingival enlargement can also be graded as:

Grade 0   -   No enlargement

Grade I   -   Confined to interdental papilla

Grade II   -   Involving papilla and marginal gingiva

Grade III   -   Covering $\geq 3/4$th of the crown of tooth.

32. IDIOPATHIC GINGIVAL ENLARGEMENT

Idiopathic gingival enlargement is a rare condition of unknown cause. In some cases, hereditary, familial and impairment of physical development may be linked.

Clinical features: The enlargement affects the attached gingiva along with marginal gingiva and interdental papilla (Fig. 4.14).

The facial and lingual surfaces of mandible and maxilla are generally affected, but may be limited to either jaw. The enlarged gingiva is pink, firm, leathery in consistency with minutely pebbled surface.

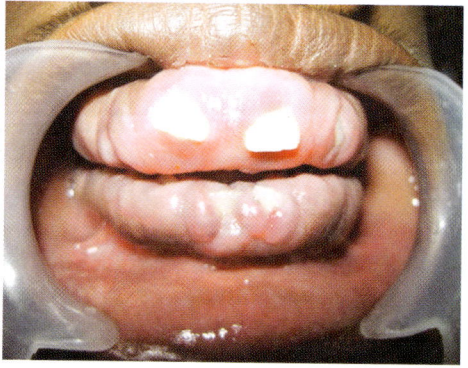

Fig. 4.14: Idiopathic gingival enlargement

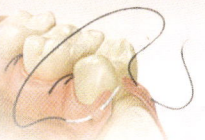
In severe cases, the teeth are almost completely covered, and the enlargement projects into the vestibule. The jaws appear distorted because of bulbous enlargement of the gingiva.

33. DILANTIN HYPERPLASIA/PHENYTOIN-INDUCED GINGIVAL ENLARGEMENT

Dilantin/phenytoin is a drug of choice for epilepsy. Dilantin hyperplasia has been reported to occur in approximately 50% of patients receiving the drug, and is more prevalent in younger patients, with no predilection for either sex or race.

Clinical features: There is gingival hyperplasia affecting especially interdental gingiva and sometimes the marginal gingiva. Gradually, the gingival changes become more diffuse, and the enlargement takes the form of a painless, discrete mass of gingival tissue that is somewhat lobulated, firm and pale pink and mulberry-shaped, resilient with no tendency to bleed. The hyperplastic gingiva gradually covers the anatomic crowns of the teeth with reduction of clinical crown. It is most prevalent in the anterior regions with the facial gingiva most frequently affected. The enlargement appears to project from beneath the gingival margin from which it is separated by a linear groove.

The primary or basic lesion starts as a painless bead-like enlargement of the facial and lingual gingival margins and interdental papillae.

Dilantin hyperplasia may occur in mouths devoid of local irritants and may be absent in mouths in which local irritants are profuse. It occurs in areas in which teeth are present and the enlargement disappears in areas from which teeth are extracted.

The presence of the enlargement makes plaque control difficult, resulting in a secondary inflammatory process that complicates the gingival hyperplasia caused by the drug. Secondary inflammatory changes add to the size of the lesion caused by dialntin, produce red or bluish red discoloration, and result in an increased tendency toward bleeding.

The enlargement is chronic and slowly increases in size until it interferes with occlusion and becomes unsightly. When surgically removed, it usually recurs, if the drug is not substituted.

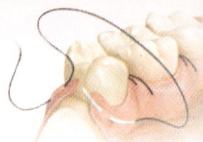

34. LEUKEMIC GINGIVAL ENLARGEMENT

The leukemia is malignancy of white blood cells characterized by:

1. Diffuse replacement of the bone marrow with proliferating leukemic cells.
2. Abnormal numbers and forms of immature white blood cells in the circulating blood.
3. Widespread infiltrates in the liver, spleen and lymph nodes.

Leukemic cells can infiltrate the gingiva and less frequently the alveolar bone. The leukemia aggravates the inflammatory process initiated by the local irritants.

Clinical Features

1. Leukemic enlargement may be diffuse or marginal, localized or generalized.
2. It may appear as diffused enlargement of the gingival mucosa, an oversized extension of the marginal gingiva, or a discrete tumor-like interproximal mass.
3. The color of gingiva is generally bluish red and has a shiny surface.
4. Consistency of gingiva is moderately firm, but there is tendency towards friability and hemorrhage, occurring either spontaneously or on slight irritation.
5. Acute painful necrotizing ulcerative inflammatory involvement may sometimes occurs.

Leukemic enlargement occurs commonly in acute and subacute types while rarely in chronic leukemia.

Histopathology

1. Various degrees of chronic inflammation with mature leukocytes and areas of connective tissue infiltrated with a dense mass of immature and proliferating leukocytes.
2. Engorged capillaries, edematous and degenerated connective tissue, epithelium with various degrees of leukocytic infiltration and edema found.
3. Isolated areas of acute necrotizing inflammation with a pseudomembranous meshwork of fibrin, necrotic epithelial cells, PMNs and bacteria are frequently seen.

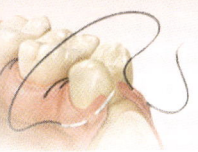

Treatment: Following consultation with the patient's physician in conjunction with appropriate medical precautions, the treatment consists of eliminating all local irritants.

35. GRANULOMA PYOGENICUM (NON-SPECIFIC CONDITIONED ENLARGEMENT/EPULIS)

It is a tumor-like gingival enlargement, which is an exaggerated conditioned response to minor trauma.

The lesion may be a discrete spherical tumor-like mass with a pedunculated attachment, to a flattened keloid-like enlargement with a broad base. It is bright red or purple and either friable or firm depending on its duration, in most of the cases it presents surface ulceration and purulent exudation.

Granuloma pyogenicum is similar in clinical and microscopic appearance to the conditioned gingival enlargement seen in pregnancy.

Histopathologically, it appears as a mass of granulation tissue with chronic inflammatory cellular infiltration. Endothelial proliferation and the formation of numerous vascular spaces are seen. The surface epithelium is atrophic or hyperplastic with surface ulcerations.

Treatment consists of removal of the lesion plus the elimination of irritating local factors (Fig. 4.15).

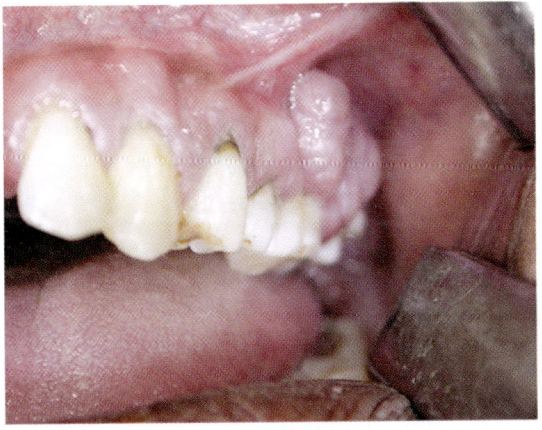

Fig. 4.15: Localized gingival enlargement

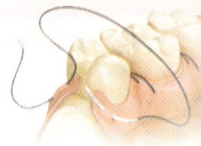

36. TREATMENT OF GINGIVAL ENLARGEMENT

1. **Chronic inflammatory enlargement:** Gingivectomy or flap operation. Scaling and root planing:
   - With pseudo pockets: Scaling and gingivoplasty
   - With true pockets: Scaling and root planing, flap surgery

2. **Abscesses:** Incision and drainage with antibiotics

3. **Drug-induced:**
   - Discontinuation and replacement of causative drug with physician's consultation.
   - Scaling and root planing.
   - Gingivoplasty or gingivectomy as required.
   - If with true pocket—undisplaced flap

4. **Leukemic gingival enlargement:**
   - Consultation with the hematologist
   - Scaling and root planing in stages
   - Systemic antibiotics before and 48 hours after each treatment.

5. **Gingival enlargement in pregnancy:**
   - Scaling and curettage
   - Surgical excision of local tumor-like enlargement, if required.

6. **Idiopathic gingival enlargement:** Surgical excision by means of gingivoplasty, gingivectomy or undisplaced flap.

7. **Gingival enlargement in puberty:** Scaling and curettage

   Treatment of all types of gingival enlargements should be reenforced with oral hygiene measures.

37. PREDISPOSING FACTORS IN ACUTE NECROTIZING ULCERATIVE GINGIVITIS (ANUG)

The specific cause of ANUG has not been established. The prevalent opinion is that it is produced by a complex of bacterial organisms but requires underlying tissue changes to facilitate the pathogenic activity of bacteria.

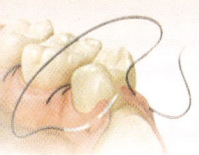

In addition to the microbiologic factors, other coincident or predisposing factors/findings, such as poor oral hygiene, injury to the gingiva and smoking, periodontal flaps, deep periodontal pockets, are common. The onset of ANUG may be promoted by the lowering of tissue resistance because of tissue insult. The disease may occur, however, in the absence of any or all of these factors.

Local predisposing factors: Pre-existing gingivitis, areas of gingiva traumatized by opposing teeth and smoking.

Debilitating diseases: Syphilis, cancer, severe gastrointestinal disorders, blood dyscrasias, and AIDS.

Oral fusospirochetal infection occasionally follows acute febrile or debilitating diseases, such as vitamin C, vitamin B and nutritional deficiencies, leukemia, agranulocytosis and erythema multiforme. Such intrinsic factors may modify the ability to resist and repair.

Psychological factors appear to be important in the etiology of ANUG. The disease often occurs in association with stressful situations. Psychologic disturbances, i.e. trait anxiety, depression and the impact of negative life events may lead to elevation of cortisol level which is associated with depression of lymphocyte and PMN function. However, the elevation may be the result rather than the cause of the ANUG.

Thus the triad of sepsis, stress and smoking are responsible for ANUG.

38. ACUTE NECROTIZING ULCERATIVE GINGIVITIS (ANUG/NUG)

A. Clinical Features

ANUG can be acute or subacute.

1. Punched out crater-like depressions at the crest of the interdental papillae extending to the marginal gingiva (Fig. 4.16).

2. The surface of the gingival craters is covered by the grey pseudomembranous slough.

3. A pronounced linear erythema demarcating the lesion from rest of the gingiva.

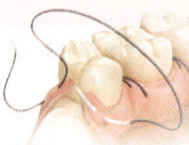

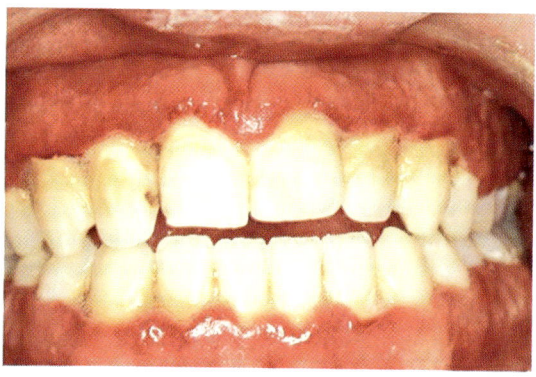

Fig. 4.16: ANUG

4. When pseudomembrane is removed, the underlying gingival margin is red, shiny and hemorrhagic.

5. Spontaneous gingival bleeding or on slightest provocation.

6. Fetid odor

7. Increased salivation.

All these clinical features are less pronounced in subacute variant.

History: Patient usually gives the history of debilitating disease, poor nutrition or sudden episode of stress.

ANUG is more common in smokers.

B. Symptoms

1. The lesions are extremely sensitive to touch, spicy and hot foods

2. Constant radiating and gnawing pain

3. "Metallic" foul taste and "pasty" saliva

4. Local lymphadenopathy

5. Fever

If untreated, ANUG can lead to necrotizing ulcerative periodontitis.

Microbiology: Following microorganisms are frequently found in ANUG lesions:

1. Spirochetes

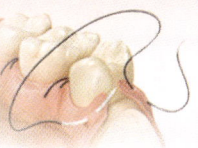

2. Fusiform bacilli
3. *Treponema microdentium*

C. Treatment

First visit:

1. Comprehensive medical history to explore current episode of stress, debilitating disease and smoking.
2. Acutely involved areas are gently cleaned with cotton rolls and dried. Topical anesthetic is applied and gently pseudomembrane is removed with wet cotton pellet.
3. Area is cleansed with warm water
4. Superficial calculus is removed.
5. Antibiotics—amoxycillin 500 mg orally four times a day for 10 days.
   Hydrogen peroxide (3%) mouthwash with equal warm water every 2 hours and/or 0.12% chlorhexidine twice daily.

Second visit: It is after 1 to 2 days of first visit. Scaling is performed, if the sensitivity permits. The patient is instructed to follow strict plaque control regimen.

Third visit: It is approximately 5 days after the second visit. Scaling and root planing are repeated, if necessary.

A patient is then re-evaluated at one month to check compliance with oral hygiene and the need for esthetic surgery which is usually needed to correct the gingival craters.

39. ACUTE HERPETIC GINGIVOSTOMATITIS (AHGS)

Acute primary herpetic gingivostomatitis is primary infection of the oral cavity caused by the herpes simplex virus (HSV) type I. It occurs most frequently in infants and children younger than 6 years of age. It is also observed in adolescents and adults, with equal frequency in males and females.

Clinical Signs

1. Diffuse erythematous, shiny involvement of gingiva along with oral mucosa.
2. Edema and gingival bleeding.

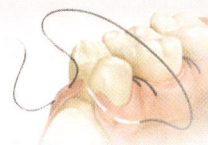

3. Discrete, spherical gray vesicles on gingiva, labial mucosa, tongue and soft palate.
4. Painful small ulcers after rupture of vesicles.

Oral Symptoms

1. Generalized soreness of the oral cavity that interferes with eating and drinking.
2. Ruptured vesicles are painful to touch.

Diagnosis

1. Established from patients history and clinical findings.
2. Laboratory test including virus culture and immunologic tests. The course of the disease is limited to 7 to 10 days.

40. ACUTE PERIODONTAL ABSCESS

Periodontal abscess is a localized purulent inflammation in the periodontal tissues. It is classified as—acute or chronic.

Acute periodontal abscess appears as an ovoid elevation of the gingiva along the lateral aspect of the root (see Fig. 3.2A). Acute abscess is usually an exacerbation of chronic inflammatory periodontal lesion. The gingiva is edematous and red, with a smooth shiny surface. The shape and consistency of the elevated area may be dome-like and relatively firm or pointed and soft. In most cases, pus may be expressed from the gingival margin by gentle digital pressure. Surrounding gingiva is enlarged, red, tender and painful. Tooth mobility may be present. Tooth is sensitive to lateral percussion. Systemic effects include malaise, fever, regional lymph node swelling and leukocytosis.

Etiology

Periodontal abscesses are associated with periodontal pockets, although these abscesses may occur in the absence of generalized periodontitis. Sudden trauma from occlusion also may be the cause. Diabetes, food impaction, overhanging margins, pushing the calculus, irritation from foreign substances, may be some of the other causes.

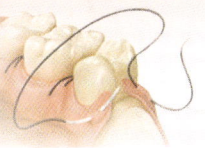
Treatment

1. Antibiotic therapy is indicated when fever or cervical lymphadenopathy is present.
2. Drainage should be established by either incising the abscess or curetting the pocket.
3. Elimination of the pocket to remove the cause of the abscess. Scaling, root planning with periodontal flap surgery can be helpful.
4. Occlusal adjustment or temporary splinting may be necessary.

41. PERICORONITIS

It is the inflammation of the gingiva in relation to the crown of an incompletely erupted tooth. The mandibular third molars are the most frequently involved. It may be acute, subacute, or chronic.

Clinical Features

The space between the partially erupted crown of the tooth and the overlying gingival flap is an ideal area for the accumulation of food debris and bacterial growth.

Acute pericoronitis is identified by involvement of the pericoronal flap and adjacent structures, as well as systemic complications (Fig. 4.17). An influx of inflammatory fluid and

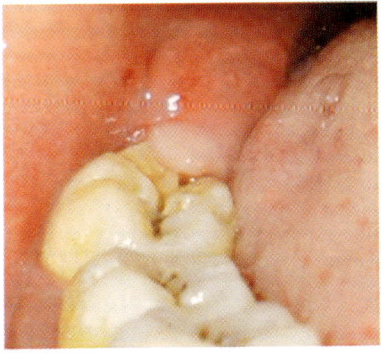

Fig. 4.17: Pericoronitis

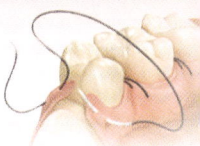

cellular exudate results in an increase in the bulk of the flap which interferes with complete closure of the jaws. The flap is traumatized by contact with the opposing jaw tooth and the inflammatory involvement is aggravated.

The clinical picture of pericoronitis:

1. Red, swollen, suppurating lesion
2. Tender and painful
3. Foul taste
4. Inability to close the mouth due to pain and swelling.
5. Fever, and malaise.
6. Pericoronal abscess, peritonsillar abscess formation, cellulites and ludwing's angina are infrequent but potential sequelae of acute pericoronitis.

Treatment consists of controlling: (i) Severity of inflammatory process, (ii) systemic complications, (iii) advisability of retaining the involved tooth.

Treatment of Acute Pericoronitis

1. Gently flushing the area with warm water to remove debris and exudates.
2. Swabbing with antiseptic after elevating the flap gently from the tooth with a scaler.
3. Prescription of antibiotics and analgesics, as required.
4. If the tooth is to be retained, pericoronal flap is removed (operculectomy).
5. Extraction is to be done to prevent the risk of bone loss around second molars.

42. CHRONIC DESQUAMATIVE GINGIVITIS

Desquamative gingivitis encompasses a variety of different oral mucous membrane diseases. The large majority of cases of so-called chronic desquamative gingivitis represent oral manifestations of one of the following dermatoses—lichen planus, mucous membrane pemphigoid, drug reactions, etc.

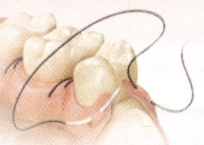

Chronic desquamative gingivitis is characterized by intense redness desquamation and ulceration of the surface epithelium of the marginal and attached gingiva.

Etiology

The cause of the conditions is unknown, and a variety of etiologic influences were suggested. The desquamative gingivitis is a nonspecific but unusual manifestation of a variety of diseases, rather than a specific disease entity.

The microscopic changes are consistent with those of underlying diseases, such as lichen planus or mucous membrane pemphigoid.

Clinical Features

I. Mild form

a. Diffuse erythema of the marginal, interdental and attached gingivae.

b. Painless condition but overall discoloration present.

c. Mostly females between 17 and 23 years age affected.

II. Moderate form

a. Patchy distribution of bright-red and gray areas involving the marginal and attached gingivae.

b. Soft, with smooth and shiny surface of gingiva.

c. Pitting on pressure and peeling of the epithelium with exposure of the underlying bleeding connective tissue on massaging with the finger is seen.

d. Occurs between 30 and 40 years of age.

e. Burning sensation and sensitivity to thermal changes seen.

f. Hard foods or tooth brushing leads to painful denudation of the gingival surface.

III. Severe form

a. Scattered, irregularly shaped areas in which the gingiva is denuded and red in appearance.

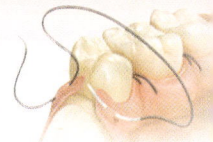

b. Gingiva separating these areas is grayish-blue, in overall appearance; the gingiva appears to be speckled.

c. The surface epithelium is friable and can be peeled off in small patches.

d. The surface vessels rupture releasing a thin aqueous fluid and exposing an underlying surface that is red and raw.

e. The mucous membrane other than the gingiva is smooth and shiny and may present a fissuring in the cheek adjacent to the line of occlusion.

f. The condition is extremely painful. The patient cannot tolerate coarse foods, condiments, or temperature changes. There is constant dry, burning sensation throughout the oral cavity.

In all forms, the lingual surface is less severely involved than the labial surface, because the tongue and friction from food excursion reduce the accumulatiosn of local irritants and limit the inflammation.

43. TREATMENT OF CHRONIC DESQUAMATIVE GINGIVITIS

1. A careful oral examination for involvement of mucous membrane or otherwise.

2. A careful history to uncover possible involvement of other mucous membranes. The presence of papular lesions of the skin on sites, such as wrists or ankles, would suggest lichen planus. Menopausal history would suggest a possible hormonal etiology.

3. Biopsy often points to the diagnosis of lichen planus or mucous membrane pemphigoid.

4. Local treatment is essential for all forms of desquamative gingivitis. Proper instruction in plaque control with oxidizing mouthwash H_2O_2 (3%) + water twice daily can be advised. The use of topical ointment and creams containing corticosteroids several times daily is also helpful.

5. Systemic therapy: The use of systemic corticosteroids with physician consultations. Prednisolone can be used in daily or every other day with dose of 30 to 40 mg in divided doses and gradually reduced to a daily maintenance dose of 5 to 10 mg or every other day.

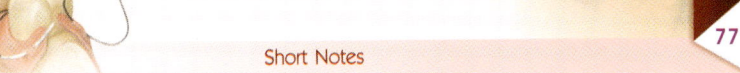

6. Hormone replacement therapy (HRT) for the lesions due to hormonal imbalance can be instituted.

44. APHTHOUS ULCER (STOMATITIS)

It is a condition characterized by depressed spherical oral ulcers.

Etiology

The etiology of apthous stomatitis is not known. Herpes simplex virus was suspected to be the cause. Other factors, suggested as causing or predisposing to apthous stomatitis, include hormonal disturbances, allergic conditions, gastrointestinal disorders and psychosomatic factors.

Clinical Features

Aphthous ulcers are characterized by well-defined, round, or ovoid, shallow ulcers with a yellowish gray central area surrounded by an erythematous halo, which heal in 7 to 10 days without scarring. The lesions may occur anywhere in the oral cavity, and are painful. It may occur as a single lesion or lesions scattered throughout the month. Aphthous ulcers can be classified as minor aphthae (<1 cm) and major aphthae (>1 cm).

Aphthous ulcers occur in the following forms:

1. Occasional aphthae is a single lesion, occurs occasionally, at intervals that vary from months to years.
2. Acute aphthae is an acute episode of aphthae, which may persist for weeks. During this period, lesions appear in different areas of the mouth. Such acute episodes are often seen in children with acute gastrointestinal disorders.
3. Chronic recurrent aphthae in which one or more oral lesions are always present. The involvement may extend over a period of years.

The treatment of aphthous stomatitis consists of elimination of the cause and nutritional supplement.

Treatment

1. Symptomatic
2. Advice nutritional supplements—protein, vitamins

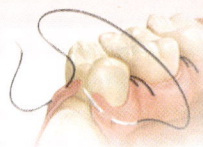

3. Advice rest
4. Topical anesthetic—lignocaine jelly 2% applied on the lesion.
5. Avoid stressful conditions.

45. CLASSIFICATION OF POCKETS

I. Depending on the destruction of the periodontal tissues, pockets can be classified as:

- **Gingival pocket** is formed by gingival enlargement without destruction of the periodontal tissues (Fig. 4.18).
- **Periodontal pocket** is formed due to destruction of the periodontal tissues (Fig. 4.19).

Periodontal pockets are further classified depending upon the position of base of the pocket with respect to alveolar crest, into two types:

1. **Suprabony**, in which base of the pocket is coronal to the underlying alveolar bone (Fig. 4.19).

2. **Infrabony**, in which base of the pocket is apical to the underlying alveolar bone (Fig. 4.20).

Infrabony pockets can be present with one-walled, two-walled or combined osseous defect.

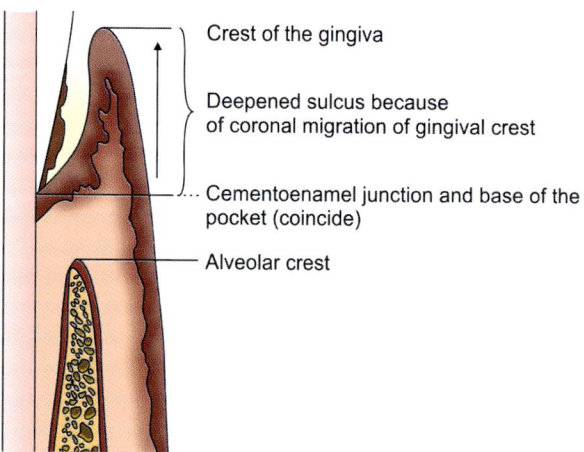

Crest of the gingiva

Deepened sulcus because of coronal migration of gingival crest

Cementoenamel junction and base of the pocket (coincide)

Alveolar crest

Fig. 4.18: Gingival (pseudo) pocket

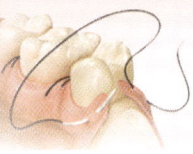

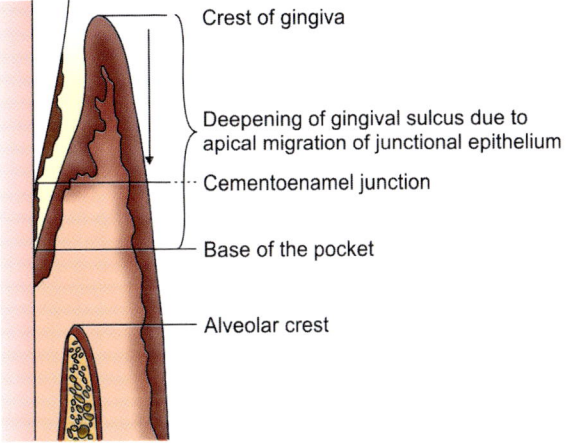

Crest of gingiva

Deepening of gingival sulcus due to apical migration of junctional epithelium

Cementoenamel junction

Base of the pocket

Alveolar crest

Fig. 4.19: Periodontal (true) pocket: Suprabony

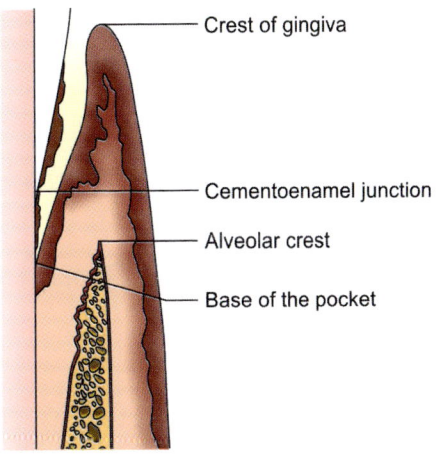

Crest of gingiva

Cementoenamel junction

Alveolar crest

Base of the pocket

Fig. 4.20: Periodontal (true) pocket: Infrabony

II. Depending upon the number of tooth surfaces involved, pockets can be:

- **Simple:** Involving only one surface.
- **Compound:** Involving more than one surface.
- **Complex and spiral:** Originating on one surface and twisting around the tooth to involve one or more additional surfaces. These types are commonly seen in furcation areas.

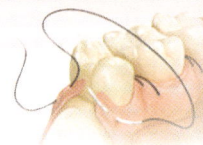

46. GINGIVAL POCKET (PSEUDO, FALSE, RELATIVE POCKET)

Pockets are of two types—1. Gingival pocket, and 2. Periodontal pocket. A gingival pocket is formed by gingival enlargement without destruction of the underlying periodontal tissues (Fig. 4.18). A gingival pocket, is a diseased gingival sulcus. The sulcus is deepened because of the increased bulk of gingiva. Gingiva covers the clinical crown and hence the clinical crowns become shorter than the anatomic crowns.

Gingival pocket may get formed due to varied reasons, viz. inflammation due to local irritants, conditions, such as puberty or pregnancy (hormonal imbalance) or drug-induced, like dilantin, nefidipine, cyclosporine.

In most of the cases, the gingival pocket responds to local treatment, i.e. scaling and polishing and certain cases require gingivoplasty, i.e. recontouring the gingiva by surgical intervention.

47. PERIODONTAL POCKET AS HEALING LESIONS

Periodontal pockets are long-standing chronic inflammatory lesions and are constantly undergoing repair. The destructive and constructive changes are going on continuously. Complete healing does not occur because of the presence of local irritants. These irritants stimulate fluid and cellular exudates, which causes degeneration of the new tissue formed in the continuous effort of repair. The balance between destructive and constructive changes determines clinical features of the pocket wall. The pocket wall may be edematous or fibrotic depending upon the inflammatory fluid and cellular exudates.

If the inflammatory fluid and exudates predominate, the pocket wall is bluish red, soft, spongy with smooth shiny surface generally referred as edematous pocket wall and when there is predominance of newly formed connective tissue cells and fibers it is referred as fibrotic pocket wall.

The most severe degenerative changes in periodontal pocket occur along the inner aspect. In some cases, inflammation and ulceration on the side of the pocket are walled off by fibrous tissue on the outer aspect. Hence pocket appears pink and fibrotic despite the inflammatory changes occurring within.

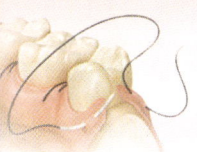

48. MICROTOPOGRAPHY OF GINGIVAL WALL OF POCKET

Interaction between host and the bacteria results in constantly changing pocket wall. Following changes have been observed.

1. **Dormant areas:** Inactive areas showing relatively flat surface with minute depressions and mounds and shedding of cells.

2. **Areas of bacterial accumulation:** Bacteria accumulate on epithelial surface, penetrating into the intercellular spaces. Types of bacteria present are cocci, rods, spirochetes and filaments.

3. **Areas of leukocyte emergence:** Leukocytes appear in the pocket wall.

4. **Areas of leukocytes–bacteria interaction:** Numerous leukocytes covered with bacteria are seen (phagocytosis).

5. **Areas of epithelial desquamation:** Which consists of various epithelial squamas, may or may not be covered with bacteria.

6. **Areas of ulceration:** This results in exposure of connective tissue.

7. **Hemorrhagic areas:** This is seen with number of erythrocytes.

49. PERIODONTAL POCKET CONTENTS

Periodontal pockets are chronic inflammatory lesions. It contains bacteria and their products, such as enzymes, toxins, and other metabolic products, gingival fluid, food remnants, salivary mucin, desquamated epithelial cells, leukocytes and calculus covered by plaque. In the presence of pus, pocket also contains living, degenerated and necrotic leukocytes, living and dead bacteria.

50. ROOT SURFACE WALL OF PERIODONTAL POCKET

Root surface wall of the periodontal pocket often undergoes changes as follows:

1. Softening of the cemental surface, which is painful during probing as a result of the exposure of the underlying dentin.

2. Microscopic areas of collagen degradation are observed.

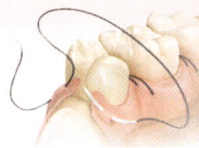

3. Bacterial products, such as endotoxins are also detected from the root surface wall.

4. Areas of increased mineralization are noted, may be due to exchange of minerals at the cementum–saliva interface.

5. Areas of demineralization are often related to the root caries.

51. PATHOGENESIS OF POCKET FORMATION

The pathological deepening of a gingival sulcus is a periodontal pocket. The changes involved are associated with different proportions of bacterial cells in dental plaque. Initially, it was assumed that bacterial attack and action was the cause for periodontal tissue destruction. Recently, it is established that the host's immunoinflammatory response to the persistent bacterial attack leads to collagen and bone destruction. This is because of various cytokines. Collagenases and other enzymes secreted by various cells in healthy and inflamed tissue, such as fibroblasts, PMNs, and macrophages destroy collagen, and these enzymes that degrade collagen and other macromolecules into small peptide are termed as matrix metalloproteinases (MMPs).

The fibroblasts phagocytize collagen fibers and degrade the inserted collagen fibrils and the fibrils of the cementum matrix. As a result of collagen loss, the apical cells of the junctional epithelium proliferate along the root. As a result of inflammation, PMNs invade junctional epithelium in increasing number ($\geq 60\%$) thereby loosing cohesiveness of epithelium leading to detachment from the root surface. Degenerative changes in the junctional epithelium at the base of pockets are less severe than those in epithelium of lateral wall of the pocket. Because migration of junctional epithelium requires healthy and viable cells, it is assumed that the degenerative changes seen in this area occur after the junctional epithelium reaches its position on cementum. The pathological changes from sulcus to periodontal pocket create an area where plaque removal becomes difficult or impossible, and a feedback mechanism sets in or is established.

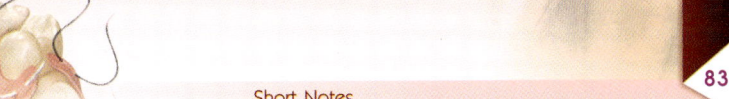
52. CLINICAL ATTACHMENT LEVEL (CAL) (PERIODONTAL ATTACHMENT LEVEL (PAL))

Measurement of clinical/periodontal attachment level (CAL/PAL) is more predictable indicator of periodontal disease than measuring the periodontal pocket.

The precise assessment and comparison of CAL/PAL at different intervals of time can determine whether attachment is being lost or gain. Gain in CAL indicates successful periodontal therapy while loss in clinical attachment shows the active lesion.

Calculation of CAL/PAL: Clinical attachment is calculated by adding the probing pocket depth to amount of gingival recession (Fig. 4.21). In the absence of gingival recession, CAL/PAL equals to the pocket depth.

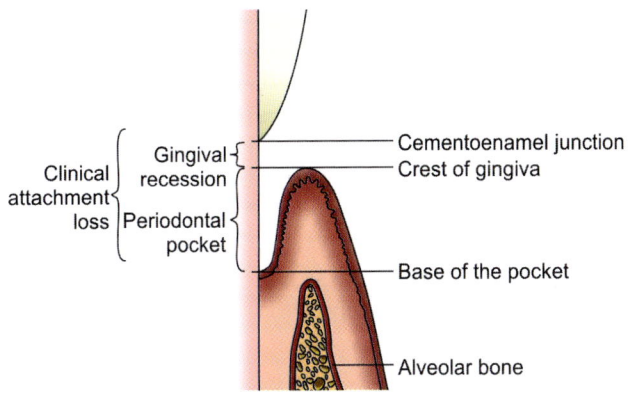

Fig. 4.21: Clinical attachment level (CAL)

53. SIGNIFICANCE OF PUS FORMATION

Pus is a common feature of periodontal disease, but only a secondary sign. Presence of pus merely reflects the nature of inflammatory changes in the pocket wall that is exudative or suppurative. It is not an indication of the severity of the destruction of the supporting tissues or the depth of the pocket. Deep pockets may exhibit little or no pus while shallow pockets may have extensive pus.

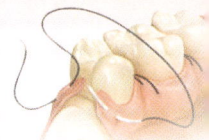

54. THE PATHWAYS OF GINGIVAL INFLAMMATION TO THE DEEP TISSUES

Gingival inflammation extends along the fiber bundles and follows the course of the blood vessels into the bone. Interproximally, inflammation spreads in the loose connective tissue around the blood vessels, through the transseptal fibers, and then into the bone through vessel channels that perforate the crest of the interdental septum. It may enter the interdental septum at the center of the crest, towards the side of the crest, or at the angle of the septum, and it may enter the bone through more than one channel. The inflammation may return from the bone into the periodontal ligament. Less frequently, inflammation spreads from the gingiva directly into the periodontal ligament and then into the interdental septum (Fig. 4.22).

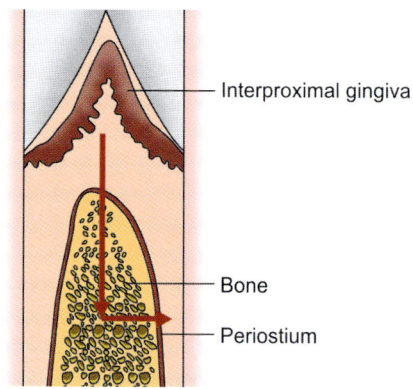

Interproximal gingiva

Bone

Periostium

Fig. 4.22: Pathways of gingival inflammation

Facially and lingually, inflammation spreads from the gingiva along the outer periosteal surface of the bone and penetrates into the marrow spaces through vessel channels in the outer cortex (Fig. 4.23).

Along its course from the gingiva to the bone, the inflammation destroys the gingival and transseptal fibers and reduces them to disorganized granular fragments among the inflammatory cells and edema. However, there is a tendency to recreate transseptal fibers across the crest of the interdental septum farther along the root as the bone destruction

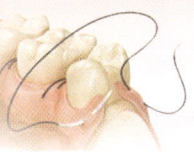

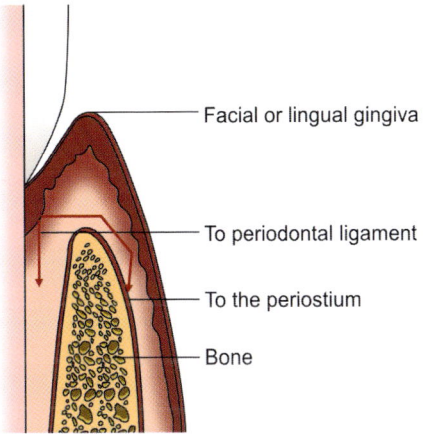

- Facial or lingual gingiva
- To periodontal ligament
- To the periostium
- Bone

Fig. 4.23: Pathways of gingival inflammation

progresses. Due to this, the transseptal fibers are present, even in cases of extreme periodontal bone loss.

The trauma from occlusion changes the pathway of gingival inflammation to the deeper periodontal tissues.

55. OSSEOUS DEFECTS IN PERIODONTAL DISEASE

Definition: An osseous defect is a concavity in the bone surrounding one or more teeth that results from periodontal disease.

The following defects may be present:

1. **Horizontal bone loss:** In this, reduction in the height of bone with margins perpendicular to the tooth surface.
2. **Vertical or angular defects:** It occurs in an oblique direction, leaving a hollowed-out trough in the bone alongside the root, the base of the defect is located apical to the surrounding bone. Angular defects are classified on the basis of the number of walls and the topography of the osseous defect. Angular defects may have one wall, two walls, or three walls (Figs 4.24A to C and 4.25). The term combined osseous defect is used when the number of walls in the apical portion of the defect may be greater than that in its occlusal portion (Fig. 4.24D). Angular defects can also

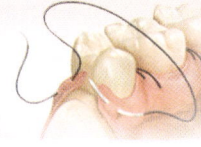

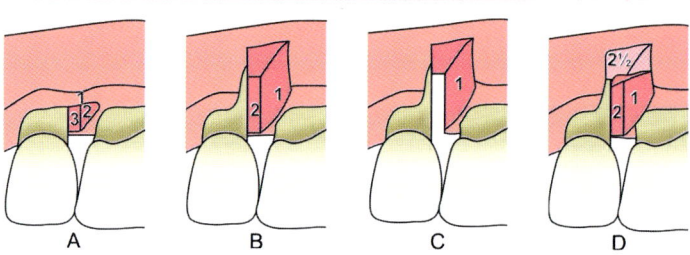

Fig. 4.24: Osseous defects: (A) Three-walled defect; (B) Two-walled defect; (C) one-walled defect; (D) Combined osseous defect

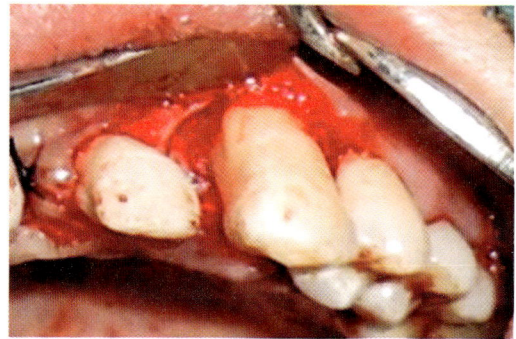

Fig. 4.25: Two-walled defect

be shallow and narrow, shallow and wide, deep and narrow, or deep and wide.

Vertical defects occurring interdentally can generally be seen on the radiograph. Surgical exposure is the only sure way to determine the presence and configuration of vertical osseous defects.

The three wall vertical defect has also been called an intrabony defect. This appears most frequently on the mesial aspects of second and third maxillary and mandibular molars. The one or two walls osseous defects are also termed as hemiseptal defects.

3. **Osseous craters:** These are concavities in the crest of the interdental bone (Fig. 4.26 A and B). Craters have been found to make up about two-thirds of all mandibular defects and one-third of all defects. They are twice as

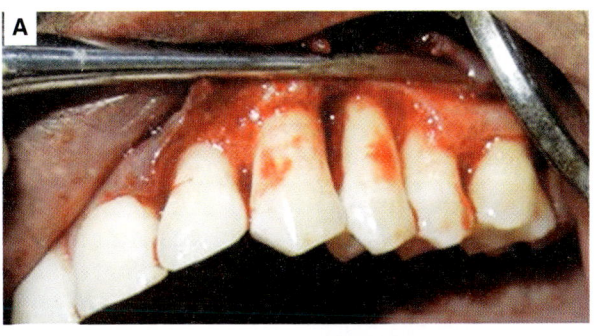

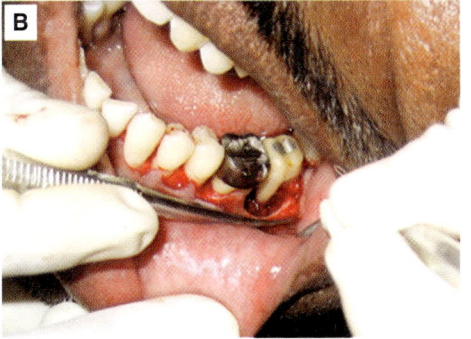

Fig. 4.26A, B: Osseous craters

common in the posterior segments as in the anterior segments. The reasons for the high frequency of interdental craters are microbial plaque and its difficulty to remove from interdental areas and the normal flat or even concave faciolingual shape of the interdental septum in mandibular molars.

The blood supply from gingiva to the center of the crest may provide a pathway for inflammation.

4. **Bulbous bone contours:** These are bony enlargements caused by exostoses, adaptation to function or buttressing bone formation.

5. **Reversed architecture/inconsistent margins:** These defects are produced due to loss of interdental bone, including the facial and/or lingual plates, without concomitant loss of radicular bone. Such defects are common in the maxilla.

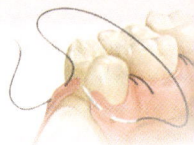

6. **Ledges:** These are plateau-like bone margins caused by resorption of thickened bony plates.

7. **Furcation involvement:** Refers to the invasion of bifurcation and trifurcation of multi-rooted teeth by periodontal disease.

8. **Dehiscences and fenestrations:** These are the bony defects in which the root is denuded of bone either complete or isolated; with or without involving marginal bone.

56. ETIOLOGY AND DIAGNOSIS OF OSSEOUS DEFECTS

Etiology

1. Plaque and calculus.
2. Occlusal trauma
3. Prolonged retention of impacted third molars.
4. Food impaction due to:
   - Open and faulty contacts.
   - Defective restoration.
   - Plunger cusp relationship.
5. Systemic disorders

Diagnosis

Periodontal disease produces different types of bone deformities or osseous defects. These are usually seen in adults. Their presence may be suggested on (a) radiographs, (b) careful probing and (c) surgical exposure of the area as are required to determine their confirmation and dimensions.

57. BUTTRESSING BONE FORMATION (LIPPING)

Bone formation when occurs to support the bony trabeculae weakened by resorption, is called as buttressing bone formation. It may be:

1. Central buttressing which occurs within the jaw
2. Peripheral buttressing occurs on the external surfaces

Due to excessive occlusal forces, bony trabeculae may get resorbed. Nature attempts to reinforce the trabeculae by forming new bone called as buttressing bone. It usually occurs

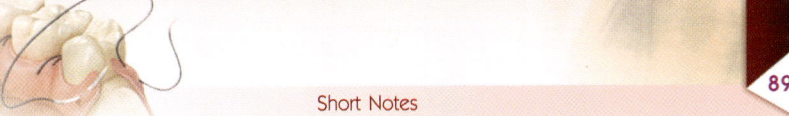

on facial or lingual alveolar surfaces. Thickening of the marginal alveolar bone is referred as lipping.

58. ETIOLOGY AND CLASSIFICATION OF INFRABONY POCKETS (ANGULAR DEFECTS)

Etiology

Inflammation is the common cause of periodontal destruction. Trauma from occlusion can produce bone destruction in the absence or presence of inflammation. The effect of occlusal forces on the periodontium is influenced by their magnitude, direction, duration and frequency.

Trauma from occlusion may alter the pathways of the extension of gingival inflammation to the underlying tissues. Inflammation then may proceed to the periodontal ligament rather than to the bone. As a result, bone loss would be angular and pockets could become infrabony. Supragingivally located plaque can become subgingival in location, if the tooth is tilted or by migration resulting in the transformation of a suprabony pocket into infrabony pocket.

In short, not every infrabony pocket develops because of a combination of trauma and inflammation, but this combination apparently increases the likelihood of a periodontal pocket becoming infrabony.

Classification

Angular defects are classified on the basis of the number of walls and the depth and width of their underlying osseous defect. Angular defects may have one wall, two walls, or three walls. The number of walls in the apical portion of the defect may be greater than that in the occlusal portion; in these cases the term combined osseous defect is used. Angular defects can also be shallow and narrow, shallow and wide, deep and narrow or deep and wide.

The three-walled vertical defect has also been termed as intrabony defect. This appears most frequently on the mesial aspects of second and third maxillary and mandibular molars. The one- or two-walled vertical defects are also called a hemiseptal defects.

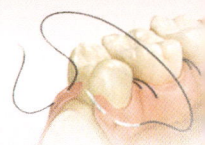

59. CLASSIFICATION OF TRAUMA FROM OCCLUSION (TFO)

I. Depending on the abruptness of change in occlusal forces, TFO can be acute or chronic.

Acute TFO: Results from abrupt occlusal impact, such as biting on a hard object.

Chronic TFO: It often develops from gradual changes in occlusion produced by tooth wear, drifting movement and extrusion of teeth, combined with parafunctional habits.

II. Depending upon the magnitude of the occlusal forces or ability of the periodontium, TFO can be primary or secondary.

Primary TFO: When it is the result of alteration in occlusal forces, e.g. high filling.

Secondary TFO: It results from reduced ability of the tissues to resist the occlusal forces (periodontitis).

60. PRIMARY TRAUMA FROM OCCLUSION

Definition: When trauma from occlusion is the result of alterations in occlusal forces which result in tissue injury, it is called as primary trauma from occlusion.

Diagnosis of primary occlusal trauma:

1. Increased tooth mobility
2. Pain
3. Food impaction
4. Fremitus test

Primary trauma from occlusion occurs, if trauma from occlusion is considered the primary etiologic factor in periodontal destruction and if the only local alteration to which a tooth is subjected is from occlusion, i.e. (i) The insertion of a "High filling", (ii) the insertion of a prosthetic replacement that creates excessive forces on abutment and antagonistic teeth, (iii) the drifting movement or extrusion of teeth into spaces, and (iv) Orthodontic movement of teeth into functionally unacceptable positions.

The changes which are observed due to primary trauma from occlusion on periodontium are severe pain, tenderness of the tooth or teeth at times, mobility of the tooth and abscess

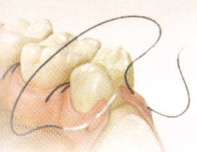

formation. At the same time, it is observed that primary trauma from occlusion does not alter the level of connective tissue attachment and does not initiate pocket formation. The changes, which are produced on the tooth and its surrounding supporting structures, are reversible when the abnormal or excessive forces or trauma is removed.

61. RESPONSE OF TISSUE TO ALTERED OCCLUSAL FORCES

Increased occlusal forces: Response of the periodontal tissue occurs in three stages which are, injury, repair and adaptive remodelling of the periodontium.

Insufficient occlusal forces: This results in atrophy of the fibers and thinning of periodontal ligament.

62. PLUNGER CUSPS

Plunger cusps are cusp points that forcibly wedge food into the interproximal spaces between opposing teeth and cause food impaction. The plunger cusp effect may occur with wear or be the result of a shift in tooth position (Fig. 4.27A). If a tooth has a prominent cusp that meets the marginal ridges of the pair of opposing teeth, it may lead to food impaction. This is especially true when the opposing teeth are mobile and the antagonist is firm. Such wedging is conducive to food impaction. The wedging cusp is termed a plunger cusp (Fig. 4.27B). The cusp points, in such cases, should be rounded

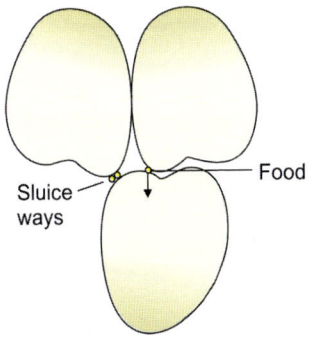

Fig. 4.27A: Normal intercuspal relation

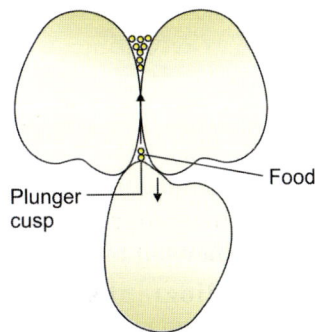

Fig. 4.27B: Plunger cusp causing food impaction

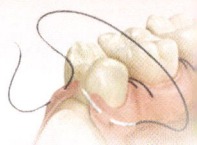

and shortened. At times it is observed that plunger cusps cause discomfort, pain or tenderness of the opposing teeth besides food impaction. In chronic or long-standing cases, interproximally, vertical bone loss takes place.

63. METHODS TO DETECT PREMATURE CONTACT

1. **Direct inspection of teeth:** During the final stages of retruded contacting adjustment, there are minute discrepancies that cause the mandible to slip in extremely small amount.

2. **Digital pressure (fremitus):** A moistened fingertip placed over the labial surfaces of the teeth while the teeth are in contact with the antagonist, vibrations can be felt (Fremitus). The determination of fremitus is not only important from a diagnostic point of view but is also most desirable means of determining an end point to the occlusal adjustment procedure.

3. **Casts:** Casts are extremely important adjunct in the oral examination. They indicate the position and inclination of the teeth, proximal contacts and view of lingual cuspal relationship.

4. **Marking paper:** The preferred paper is one that is thick and rather smudgy, gives a definitive sound when teeth strike it, and allows for comparative imprints on the paper itself that can be read as a wax bite. This is useful to locate initial interference.

5. **Wax recording:** The use of wax is an important adjunct to the study of occlusal contacts.

6. **Sound:** The sound of a properly adjusted occlusion is distinct, crisp, and clear and is caused by all teeth striking simultaneously in the correct retruded contacting position. When interference is present in closure, the sound is somewhat mushy and prolonged.

7. **Radiographs:** Radiographic changes in trauma from occlusion may indicate some changes in premature contact positions. The changes may be in the lamina dura, in the morphology of the alveolar bone, in the width of the

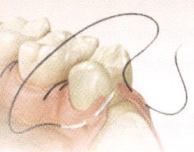

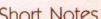

periodontal ligament space, and in the density of the surrounding cancellous bone.

64. FOOD IMPACTION

Food impaction is the forceful wedging of food into the periodontal tissues by occlusal forces. It is more common in the interproximal areas, but may occur on the facial and lingual surfaces also. Excessive anterior overbite is a very common cause of food impaction, and it aggravates the severity of pre-existent pathologic changes. Failure to recognize and eliminate, it may result in unsuccessful outcome of an otherwise thoroughly treated periodontal disease. The following signs and symptoms may occur in association with food impaction.

1. Feeling of pressure and urge to dig between the teeth.
2. Vague pain deep in the jaws.
3. Gingival bleeding, swollen gingiva and a foul taste.
4. Periodontal abscess formation
5. Gingival recession
6. Elevation of the tooth in its socket, prematurity in functional contact, and sensitivity to percussion.
7. Destruction of alveolar bone, and vertical bony defects.
8. Caries of the root

Mechanism of food impaction: Proper proximal contact, contour of the occlusal surface, marginal ridges and developmental grooves together, deflect food away from the interproximal space. After wearing down of the teeth there is loss of normal convexities which in turn leads to the wedging effect of the opposing cusp into the interproximal space and food impaction results. Forceful wedging of food into the gingiva on the facial surfaces of mandibular anteriors and palatal surfaces of maxillary anteriors produces varying degrees of periodontal involvement.

Lateral food impaction: In addition to these factors, lateral pressure from the lips, cheeks and tongue may also force food interproximally. It occurs when gingival embrasure is enlarged by tissue destruction in periodontal disease or by recession.

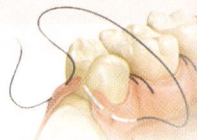

65. OCCLUSION

The relationship of maxillary and mandibular teeth when they are in functional contact during activity of the mandible is referred as occlusion.

Ideal occlusion refers to aesthetically pleasing and physiologically stable. It includes functional and neuro-muscular harmony as well as stability of masticatory system.

Physiologic occlusion: It does not show the signs of occlusion related pathosis.

Balanced occlusion: It is an occlusion in which balanced and equal contacts are maintained throughout the entire arch during all excursions of the mandible.

Traumatic occlusion: An occlusion judged to be causative factor for periodontal tissue injury.

Trauma from occlusion: It is the periodontal tissue injury caused by traumatic occlusion.

Therapeutic occlusion: It is the type of occlusion achieved after specific interventions to correct the dysfunction.

Malocclusion: Malalignment of teeth.

Malocclusion is not always traumatic but the clinically apparently normal occlusion can be a traumatic one. Hence in periodontal diagnosis and treatment, traumatic occlusion is important.

66. PATHOLOGICAL MIGRATION OF TEETH

It refers to tooth displacement or migration that results when the balance among the factors that maintain physiologic tooth position is disturbed by periodontal disease.

Pathologic migration (Fig. 4.28) is seen most frequently in the anterior region, but posterior teeth may also be affected. Migration is usually accompanied by mobility and rotation of teeth. Pathologic migration in the occlusal direction is termed extrusion.

Two factors play a role in maintaining the normal position of the teeth: (i) The health and normal height of the perio-dontium, and (ii) the forces exerted on the teeth.

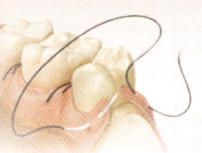

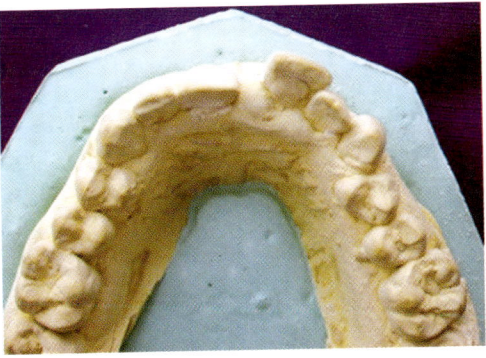

Fig. 4.28: Pathological migration

Pathologic migration, therefore, occurs under conditions that weaken the periodontal support.

The inflammatory destruction of the periodontium in periodontitis creates an imbalance between the forces maintaining the tooth in position and the occlusal and muscular forces.

The tooth with weakened support is unable to maintain its normal position in the arch and moves away from the opposing force, unless it is restrained by proximal contact. As its position changes, the tooth is subjected to abnormal occlusal forces, which aggravate the periodontal destruction and tooth migrates.

Pathologic migration may continue after a tooth no longer contacts its antagonist, pressure from the tongue, food bolus during mastication, and from proliferating granulation tissue, provides the force.

Pathologic migration is also an early sign of localized aggressive periodontitis wherein drifting of maxillary and mandibular teeth with diastema is observed.

Changes in the forces exerted on the teeth: Changes in the magnitude, the direction, the frequency of the forces exerted on the teeth can induce pathologic migration if the periodontium is sufficiently weakened. Changes in the forces may result from unreplaced missing teeth or trauma from occlusion.

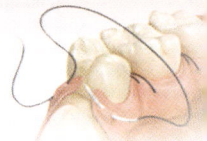

67. INDICATIONS FOR OCCLUSAL ADJUSTMENT (CORONOPLASTY)

The rationale of occlusal adjustment is based upon the fact that tissue injury caused by unfavorable occlusal forces is reversible and will undergo repair when forces are corrected. In general, occlusal adjustment (coronoplasty) is not often indicated in periodontal therapy except when a patient has occlusion weakened by bone loss.

Occlusal adjustment is indicated under the following conditions:

1. In patients with trauma from occlusion. Periodontal response rather than the presence or absence of pre-maturities determines whether an occlusion is traumatic. The periodontal injury manifested in the form of excessive tooth mobility, angular thickening of the periodontal ligament, vertical bone loss, furcation involvement, migration of maxillary anterior teeth and occlusal wear.

2. In patients with periodontal support reduced by perio-dontal disease, the capacity of the teeth to withstand occlusal forces is reduced. The occlusion is adjusted to eliminate the occlusal forces that might overburden the already weakened periodontium. (This is done after the complete treatment of weakened periodontium.)

3. In patients with TMJ disorders or muscle disturbances caused by occlusal disharmony.

4. In patients with parafunctional habits, where it is likely that the trauma from occlusion is caused more by repetitive parafunctional forces.

5. Planned occlusal reconstruction

68. CORONOPLASTY (OCCLUSAL ADJUSTMENT)

The coronoplasty is the selective reduction of occlusal areas with the primary aim of influencing the mechanical contact relationship. The correction of occlusal supracontact is necessary so as to create smooth closure of cusps into fossa and marginal ridges.

The correction of occlusal supracontacts consists of:

1. Grooving

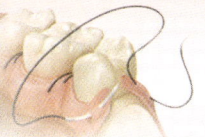

2. Spheroiding
3. Pointing.

1. **Grooving:** This is performed with a tapered cutting stones. In this, the depth of developmental grooves is restored until a desired depth is attained.

2. **Spheroiding:** It consists of reducing the supracontact while restoring the original tooth contour. Starting 2 to 3 mm mesial and/or distal to the prematurity, the tooth is recontoured from the occlusal margin to a distance 2 to 3 mm apical to the supracontact. This is done with a light "paint brush" stroke with preserving the occlusal height of the cusps.

3. **Pointing:** It consists of restoring cusp point contours by reshaping the tooth with rotating cutting tools.

Coronoplasty can be accomplished using a variety of different sequences, if the correction is of few teeth or step by step.

69. CHRONIC PERIODONTITIS (ADULT PERIODONTITIS)

It is an infectious disease resulting in inflammation within the supporting tissues of the teeth, progressive attachment and bone loss.

Clinical Features

Signs

1. Associated diseases, usually becomes significant in the mid-thirties or later.
2. Supragingival and subgingival plaque and calculus present.
3. Gingival inflammation; loss of stippling.
4. Pocket formation
5. Loss of periodontal attachment
6. Loss of alveolar bone (seen radiographically)
7. Occasional suppuration
8. Predilection for interproximal areas
9. Rate of disease progression is usually slow but may be modified by systemic and environmental factors.

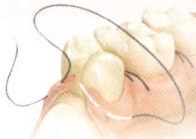

Symptoms

1. Bleeding gums while brushing or eating, spacing occurs between teeth as a result of tooth movement usually painless.
2. Occasionally sensitivity to heat, cold or both because of exposed roots.
3. Patient may feel localized dull pain, sometimes radiating deep into the jaw.
4. The presence of areas of food impaction may add to the patient's discomfort.
5. Gingival tenderness or "itchiness" may also be found.

Classification of Chronic Periodontitis

I. **Depending upon the number of sites involved:**
   a. **Localized periodontitis:** Less than 30% of the sites assessed in mouth demonstrate attachment loss and bone loss.
   b. **Generalized periodontitis:** 30% or more of the sites assessed in the mouth demonstrate attachment loss and bone loss.

II. **Depending upon the severity of the disease:**
   a. **Slight (mild) periodontitis:** 1 to 2 mm of clinical attachment loss has occurred.
   b. **Moderate periodontitis:** 3 to 4 mm of clinical attachment loss has occurred.
   c. **Severe periodontitis:** >5 mm clinical attachment loss has occurred.

Disease progression: Chronic periodontitis does not progress at an equal rate in all affected sites throughout the mouth.

Etiology

1. Prior history of periodontal disease.
2. Local factors: Plaque accumulation on tooth and gingival surfaces at the dentogingival junction is considered the primary initiating agent.

3. Potential local factors: Overhanging margins of restorations, root caries, furcation involvements, crowded and mala-ligned teeth, root grooves and concavities.
4. Systemic factors, e.g. diabetes, hormonal imbalance.
5. Environmental factors, e.g. smoking.
6. Behavioral factors, e.g. stress.
7. Genetic factors.

70. NECROTIZING ULCERATIVE PERIODONTITIS (NUP)

Two types of NUP have been described according to their relationship with AIDS.

a. **Non-AIDS/HIV-associated necrotizing ulcerative perio-dontitis:** This form of periodontitis usually follows long-term repeated episodes of untreated or incompletely treated ANUG, which is characterized by areas of ulceration and necrosis of the gingival margin forming pseudomembrane. The ulcerated margin is surrounded by an erythematous halo. The lesions are painful and bleed often, giving rise to localized lymphadenopathy and even fever and malaise. The repeated insults to the periodontium causes destruction of the interproximal tissues leaving inter-proximal crater formation in both soft tissue and alveolar bone (Fig. 4.29). Necrotizing ulcerative perio-dontitis is characterized by deep interdental osseous craters, but deep conventional pockets are not found, because the ulcerative and necrotizing character of the gingival lesion destroys the junctional epithelium, removing the mechanisms of pocket deepening.

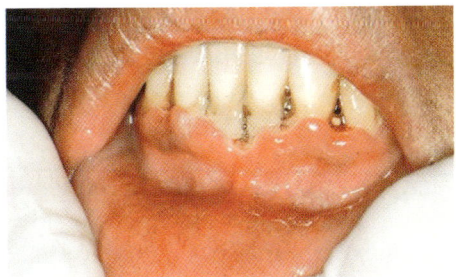

Fig. 4.29: Necrotizing ulcerative periodontitis

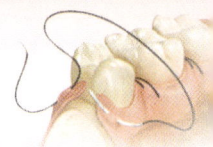

Lesions of NUP can lead to severe bone loss, tooth mobility, and tooth loss. Etiology of NUP is thought to be impaired bactericidal activity of PMNs and same as ANUG.

b. **AIDS/HIV-associated necrotizing ulcerative periodontitis:** Gingival and periodontal lesions are frequently found in patients with HIV infection or AIDS. These lesions in HIV positive patients appear to be similar to those seen in NUP in HIV negative patients, but frequently result in complications that are rare in non-AIDS patients and more destructive. These complications are soft tissue necrosis with exposure of bone and sequestration of bone fragments, extending to the vestibular, palatal areas and becoming necrotizing ulcerative stomatitis. Generalized NUP may be present after severe depletion of CD4+ cell counts.

Etiology of AIDS associated NUP: Opportunistic infections are present favored by AIDS:

a. *Candida albicans*

b. Higher prevalence of *A. actinomycetemcomitans*, *P. intermedia*, *P. gingivalis*, *F. nucleatum* and *Campylobacter spp.*

Treatment consists of gentle debridement and scaling and root planing. Meticulous oral hygiene must be established including antimicrobial mouthrinses.

71. LOCALIZED AGGRESSIVE PERIODONTITIS (LAP, LOCALIZED JUVENILE PERIODONTITIS)

LAP, formerly classified as localized juvenile periodontitis, refers to a relatively uncommon form of periodontitis usually has an age of onset at about puberty. It is characterized by rapid alveolar bone destruction in connection with first molars and incisors; with minimal signs or no clinical signs of gingival inflammation.

Clinical Features

During the early phases, the disease is frequently not recognized because the gingiva appears to be healthy. Distolabial migration of the maxillary incisors with diastema formation is a frequent finding. Minimal amount of plaque and calculus are seen during the early phases of the disease (Fig. 4.30).

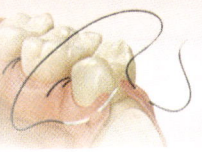

Both males and females are affected by this disease while higher incidence was reported in females.

Classic sign is lack of clinical inflammation, despite the presence of deep periodontal pockets, mobility of molars, dull pain, sensitivity and formation of periodontal abscess.

Etiology

Not known. Although the quantity of plaque may be limited, it often contains elevated levels of *A. actinomycetemcomitans* and *Porphyromonas gingivalis*. Functional defects of PMNs and monocytes were also noted.

Reasons for limitation of periodontal destruction to certain teeth:

1. After the initial attack on the incisors and first molars (i.e. the first permanent teeth to erupt) adequate immune defenses are stimulated to produce opsonizing antibodies against *Aggregatibacter actinomycetemcomitans* (A.a).

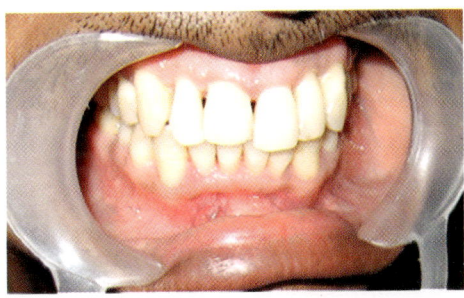

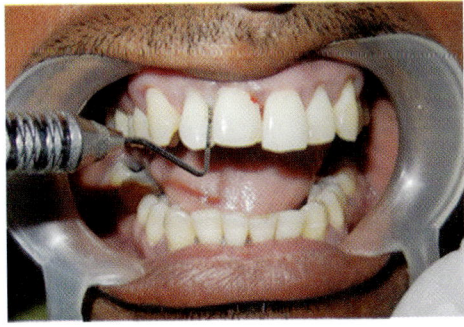

Fig. 4.30: Clinical picture of aggressive periodontitis

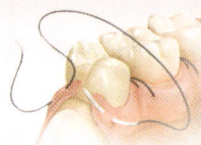

2. Bacteria antagonistic to *A. actinomycetemcomitans* develop and decrease destructiveness of the lesion.

3. *A. actinomycetemcomitans* loses its leukotoxin producing capacity for unknown reasons. If this happens, the disease may get arrested.

4. Defect in cementum formation may be responsible for localization of these lesions.

Burnout of the disease: Localized forms of aggressive periodontitis have been known to arrest spontaneously. This unexplained curtailment of disease progression has sometimes been referred to as a burnout of the disease.

Radiographic signs: Angular or vertical alveolar bone loss occurs around the permanent first molars and incisors. An arch-shaped bone loss extends from the distal of second premolar to the mesial of second molar. Bilateral bone loss is common (mirror image).

Treatment

Conventional periodontal therapy:
- Scaling and root planing
- Osseous resective surgery
- Regenerative therapy

Antimicrobial Therapy
- Systemic administration of antibiotics: Doxycycline is promising against A.a.
- **Local drug delivery**
- **Full mouth disinfection**
- **Host modulation**

72. FULL MOUTH DISINFECTION

This concept was introduced by Quirynen et al referred to the procedure of full mouth debridement completed in two appointments within 24 hours. This consists of scaling and root planing, brushing of tongue with chlorhexidine gel (1%) for one

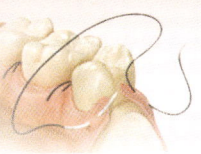

minute, rinsing of mouth with a chlorhexidine solution (0.2%) for two minutes and irrigation of periodontal pocket with chlorhexidine solution (1%).

The treatment modality was found to be effective in chronic periodontitis with respect to reduction in probing depth, especially in deep (7–8 mm) pockets. It was also shown to be effective in aggressive periodontitis in terms of clinical attachment gain and for longer periods the results were stable.

73. REFRACTORY PERIODONTITIS

It is a condition in which multiple sites in patient exhibit continued attachment loss inspite of usual and customary periodontal therapy. Patients that, for unknown reasons, do not respond to treatment and/or recur soon after adequate treatment; have been referred to as refractory periodontitis. It should be distinguished from recurrent disease in which the irritants were never completely removed, and the disease may temporarily have become less severe but never resolved.

Clinical features: Refractory periodontitis occurs either by new involvement of the additional teeth or by increased bone loss and attachment loss in previously treated sites with bleeding and suppuration.

Etiology

1. Abnormal host response
2. Resistant micro-organisms
3. Untreatable morphologic problems or combinations of any of these

    Two types of refractory periodontitis:

    a. Refractory sites where anatomic conditions prevent complete plaque removal. This is a most common form.
    b. Cases of aggressive periodontitis including prepubertal form and various syndromes.

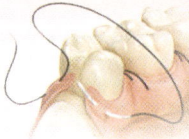

74. ETIOLOGY OF PERIODONTAL DISEASE

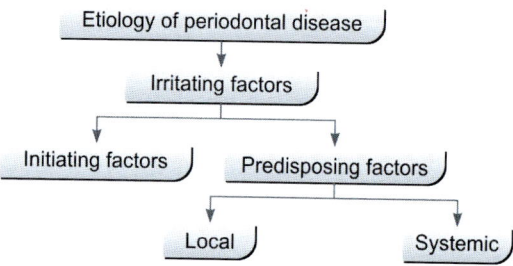

Initiating factors: Bacterial plaque

Predisposing Factors

Local

- Materia alba
- Food debris
- Dental stains
- Calculus, caries
- Smoking and tobacco consumption
- Food impaction
- Iatrogenic factors
- Dental morphological defects, poor or improper oral hygiene.
- Soft and sticky food
- Mouth breathing.

Systemic

- Endocrine: Puberty, pregnancy, menopause
- Nutritional disorders and deficiencies:
  - Vitamin deficiencies, protein deficiencies, malnutrition
- Drugs:
  - Antiepileptic drug, such as dilantin sodium
  - Antihypertensive, such as nifedipine
  - Immunosuppressant, such as cyclosporine
  - Contraceptive medications.
- Environmental factors: Smoking
- Behavioural factors: Stress

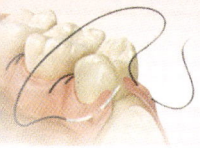

- Hereditary and genetic anomalies
- Metabolic disease: Diabetes mallitus.
- Hematological disturbances: Leukemia, anemia, etc.

75. DENTAL PLAQUE

Definition

Dental plaque is defined as a structured resilient yellow-grayish deposit that adheres tenaciously to the tooth surface and other hard surfaces of the oral cavity including removable and fixed restorations.

Classification

A. **Supragingival:** Found at or above the gingival margin
B. **Subgingival:** Found below the gingival margin, between the tooth and the gingival pocket epithelium (Fig. 4.31).
   1. **Tooth-associated:** Associated with tooth surface and attached
   2. **Tissue-associated:** Associated with soft tissue, and unattached.

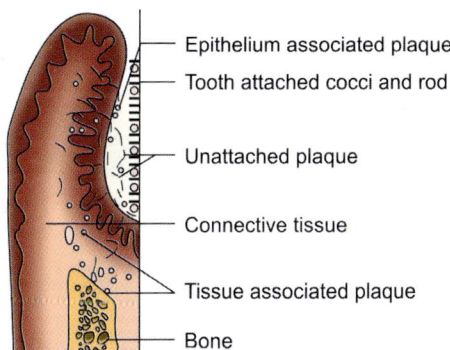

Fig. 4.31: Classification of subgingival plaque

Composition

a. Intercellular matrix
   1. Organic content.
   2. Inorganic content.
      - **Organic contents:** Polysaccharides, proteins, glyco-proteins and lipid material.

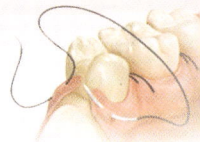

- **Inorganic contents:** Primarily calcium and phosphorus and trace amounts of sodium, potassium and fluoride.
b. Proliferating microorganisms, scattered epithelial cells, leukocytes, macrophages, mycoplasma, yeast, protozoa and viruses.

76. FORMATION OF DENTAL PLAQUE

It occurs in three stages:

I. **Formation of dental pellicle:** Pellicle forms by selective adsorption of the environmental macromolecules. Mechanisms involved in enamel pellicle formation include electrostatic, van der Waals and hydrophobic forces. The hydroxyapatite surface has a predominance of negatively charged phosphate groups that interact directly or indirectly with positively charged components or salivary and crevicular fluid macromolecules.

Pellicle provides a substrate to which bacteria in the environment attach.

II. **Initial colonization and adhesion to the tooth surface:** The initial bacteria colonizing the pellicle-coated tooth surface are predominantly gram-positive facultative microorganisms, like *Actinomyces* and *Streptococcus spp.*

These colonizers adhere to the pellicle through specific molecules called "adhesins" on the bacterial surface that interact with receptors in dental pellicle.

For example: *A. viscosus* possesses fibrous protein structures called fimbriae which bind to protein rich proteins in the dental pellicle resulting in the attachment of bacteria to pellicle.

As plaque matures, there is a transition from the early aerobic environment characterized by gram-positive facultative species to a highly oxygen deprived environment in which gram-negative anaerobic microorganisms predominate.

III. **Secondary colonization and plaque maturation:** Secondary colonizers including *Prevotella intermedia, Prevotella loescheii, Capnocytophaga* species, *Fusobacterium nucleatum* and *P. gingivalis* adhere to cells of bacteria already present

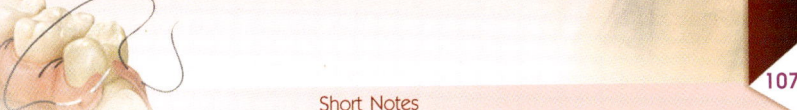

in the plaque mass. Different species and genera of plaque microorganisms adhere to one another by a process known as coaggregation or coadhesion. This leeds to the development of microcolonies and eventually to a mature biofilm.

77. PLAQUE MICROBIOTA AND THEIR ACTIONS

Following are genera of microorganisms representative of the numerous bacteria that are related to the plaque microbiota.

1. Gram-positive cocci, e.g. *Streptococcus, Staphylococcus.*
2. Gram-positive rods, e.g. *Lactobacillus, Actinomyces.*
3. Gram-negative rods, e.g. *Bacteroides, Fusobacterium*
4. Spirochetes

Microorganisms in the plaque exert their destructive action, causing tissue injury, damage and disease by various mechanisms

1. Production of toxins—exotoxins and endotoxins
2. Production of enzymes—collagenase and proteases
3. Bacterial antigens
4. Bacterial waste products—ammonia, hydrogen sulfide.

All these microbial products act as irritating substances that produce the changes in the periodontal tissues.

Bacterial penetration into the periodontium may be an important factor in the pathogenesis of periodontal disease.

78. NON-SPECIFIC AND SPECIFIC PLAQUE HYPOTHESIS

Non-specific plaque hypothesis: Previously, it was believed that entire plaque flora and its noxious products are responsible for the periodontal disease. This concept, termed as 'non-specific plaque hypothesis' put forward by W. Loesche in 1976.

But it was contradicted by following facts:

1. Some individuals, inspite of having considerable amount of plaque only few developed gingivitis but never developed periodontitis.
2. Conversely, individuals with periodontitis presented with considerable site specificity.

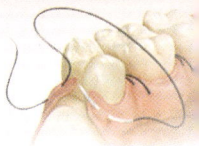

Therefore, W. Loesche himself presented the concept of specific plaque hypothesis.

Specific plaque hypothesis: It states that only certain plaque is pathogenic and its pathogenicity depends on the presence of or increase in number of specific microorganisms. Specific plaque hypothesis was accepted well when *A. actinomycetemcomitans* was identified as pathogen in localized aggressive periodontitis.

However, periodontal therapy still depends on control of plaque accumulation and focuses on removal of local irritants which is based on non-specific plaque hypothesis, or ecologic plaque hypothesis.

79. MICROBIOLOGY OF PERIODONTAL POCKET

Pocket formation starts as an inflammatory change in the connective tissue wall of the gingival sulcus caused by microbial plaque. The cellular and fluid inflammatory exudate causes degeneration of the surrounding connective tissue, including gingival fibers. Bacterial invasion of the apical and lateral areas of the pocket wall occurs in chronic periodontitis. Filaments, rods and coccoid organisms with predominant gram-negative, microbes have been found in intercellular spaces of the epithelium. Bacteria invade the intercellular space initially under exfoliating epithelial cells, but they are also found between deeper epithelial cells and accumulating on the basement lamina. The presence of bacteria has also been reported within the oral epithelium and adjacent connective tissue of deep periodontal pockets. This may occur in nonkeratinized inflamed areas of the gingiva.

Periodontal pocket, the hallmark of periodontitis is found in all types of periodontitis. Bacteria associated with each type are as follows:

I. **Chronic periodontitis:** *P. intermedia, C. rectus, P. gingivalis, T. forsythia, E. corrodens, A. actinomycetemcomitans, Treponema,* etc. (active sites).

II. **Localized aggressive periodontitis:** Gram-negative, capnophilic anaerobic rods, *A. actinomycetemcomitans*

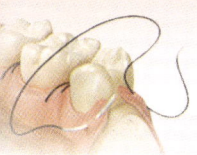

(90%), *P. gingivalis. E. corrodens, C. rectus, F. nucleatum, capanocytophaga* and *Spirochetes.*

III. Aggressive periodontitis: Same as above. High proportion of *P. gingivalis, P. intormedia* and *Treponema.*

80. HOST MICROBIAL INTERACTIONS IN PERIODONTAL DISEASE

Destruction of the tissue in periodontal disease involves a complex interplay between periodontal pathogens and host tissues. Periodontal pathogens such as *P. gingivalis, A. actinomycetemcomitans, T. forsythia, F. nucleatum. C. rectus, P. micros* and *E. corrodens,* are responsible for tissue destruction.

These microorganisms evade the first level of host defense and manage to adhere to the tooth surface, tissue or pre-existing plaque by either bacterial adhesion or substrate receptors.

Once established adherence, these bacteria invade further host defense mechanism by one or more of the following ways:

1. Degrading the specific antibody, e.g. *P. gingivalis*
2. Altering the PMN function, e.g. *A. actinomycetemcomitans*
3. Affecting the inflammatory mediators
4. Production of certain enzymes, such as collagenase, trypsin, like enzymes, etc., which are capable of degrading host tissues; along with the toxins.

This results in destruction of periodontal tissues which in turn favor the accumulation of more periodontal pathogens and thus leading to progressive periodontal disease.

81. SUBGINGIVAL MICROBIAL COMPLEXES

Molecular identification techniques, such as; DNA hybridization methodology divided 40 subgingival microorganisms into different color-coded complexes that are found together in health or disease. These are group of microorganisms frequently found in clusters and color-coded for easy conceptualization.

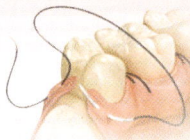

Early Colonizers

a. Yellow complex:
Streptococcus sp.

b. Purple complex:
A. odontolyticus

Secondary Colonizers

a. Green complex: Periodontal pathogens
E. corrodens,
A. actinomycetemcomitans,
Capnocytophaga spp.

b. Orange complex: Periodontal pathogens
Fusobacterium
Prevotella
Campylobacter spp

c. Red complex: Associated with bleeding on probing
P. gingivalis
T. forsythia
T. denticola

Presence of these complexes indicates the microbial interdependency in plaque biofilm.

82. GINGIPAINS

Gingipains are multifunctional proteins that play a role in adhesion, tissue degradation and evasion of the host response. These are cysteine proteases secreted by a potent perio-dontopathogen *Porphyromonas gingivalis* which are responsible for degradation of cytokines thereby down regulating the host response. Thus, gingipains are important virulence factors of *P. gingivalis*, and are likely to be associated with the development of periodontitis.

It is, therefore, suggested that gingipains inhibition by new generation antibiotic—gingipain specific inhibitor—can be helpful in the treatment of periodontitis caused by *P. gingivalis* infection.

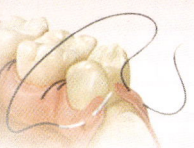

83. DENTAL CALCULUS

Definition: Dental calculus is an adherent calcified or calcifying mass that forms on the surfaces of natural teeth.

The role of calcified deposits on teeth as a primary etiologic factor in inflammatory periodontal disease has been demonstrated by clinical research. Although dental microbial plaque has been demonstrated to be a major initiating factor in the development of gingivitis, the presence of dental calculus is of equal concern to the therapist.

When dental plaque calcifies, the resultant deposit is called dental calculus. These calcified deposits occur as hard, firmly adhering masses on the clinical crown of teeth. The surface of dental calculus is always covered with uncalcified plaque. This coating consists of micro-organisms of many types, desquamated epithelial cells and leukocytes that have migrated through the sulcular epithelium all held together by a sticky matrix.

Calculus is rough, porous and attracts more plaque. It is always covered by a microbial plaque. Calculus is permeable and may store toxic products. Hence calculus may be harmful both physically and chemically.

84. COMPOSITION OF CALCULUS

A. Inorganic content—70–90%
   a. Calcium phosphate
   b. Calcium carbonate
   c. Magnesium phosphate, and metals.

Two-thirds of inorganic component is crystalline in structure and consists of 4 main crystal forms:

- Hydroxyapatite—58%
- Magnesium whitlockite—21%
- Octacalcium phosphate—12%
- Brushite—9%

B. Organic content
   a. Protein—polysaccharide complexes.
   b. Desquamated epithelial cells.

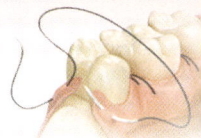

   c. Leukocytes.

   d. Microorganisms.

Content of supra- and subgingival calculus is similar except that subgingival calculus has more magnesium whitlockite and less brushite and octacalcium phosphate.

85. SUPRAGINGIVAL AND SUBGINGIVAL CALCULUS

Calculus may be classified clinically as supragingival and subgingival. This classification refers to the location the calculus at examination time.

Supragingival (salivary) calculus is located coronal to the gingival margin and most abundant opposite to the openings of salivary glands, that is on the oral surfaces of the mandibular anterior teeth and the buccal surfaces of the maxillary first molars. Supragingival calculus is creamy white or yellowish in color unless it is stained by tobacco or other pigments, with clay-like consistency (Fig. 4.32).

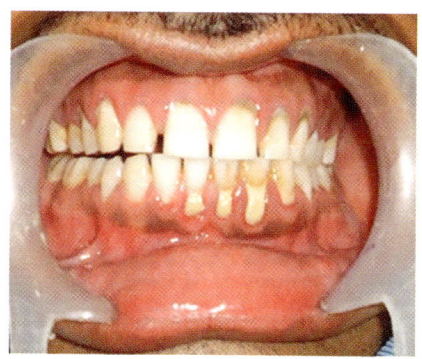

Fig. 4.32: Supragingival calculus

Subgingival (serumal) calculus may be found on any tooth in the mouth and in any periodontal pocket. Subgingival calculus is more dense than supragingival. Subgingival calculus is located below the crest of marginal gingiva. It is usually dark brown to black and is found as a concretion on the root surface of the tooth in a periodontal pocket (Fig. 4.33).

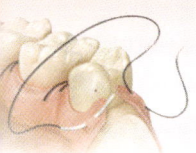

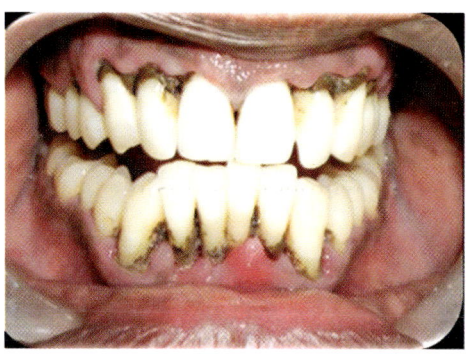

Fig. 4.33: Subgingival calculus

Clinical significance of calculus: Calculus is not the principal irritant but a significant contributing factor. Instead of irritating the gingiva directly, it provides a fixed nidus for continued accumulation of plaque and keeping it in close contact with the gingiva. It thus initiates gingival inflammation, which starts pockets formation and periodontal disease.

86. THEORIES REGARDING CALCULUS FORMATION (MINERALIZATION)

Theories regarding the mechanism whereby plaque is mineralized fit into two concepts.

1. **According to the first concept:** A rise in pH of saliva causes precipitation of calcium and phosphate salts, (a) The pH may be elevated by the loss of CO_2 and by formation of ammonia by dental plaque bacteria. (b) Colloidal proteins in saliva bind calcium and phosphate ions and maintain a supersaturated solution. With stagnation of saliva, colloids settle out leading to precipitation of calcium and phosophate salts. (c) Phosphatase liberated from dental plaque, desquamated epithelial cells or bacteria precipitates calcium phosphate by hydrolyzing organic phosphates in saliva, thus increasing the concentration of free phosphate ions. (d) Esterase (enzyme) may initiate calcification.

2. **According to the second concept:** Seeding agents induce small foci of calcification which enlarge and coalesce to

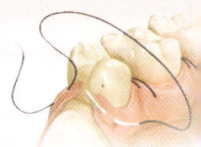
form calcified mass (also referred as epitactic concept or heterogeneous nucleation). The carbohydrate protein complex may initiate calcification by removing calcium from the saliva (chelation) and binding with it to form nuclei that induce subsequent deposition of minerals. Plaque bacteria have also been implicated as possible seeding agents. Filamentous organisms, bacteroids and *Veillonella* species have the ability to form intracellular apatite crystals. Calculus formation spreads until the matrix and bacteria are calcified.

87. MODES OF ATTACHMENT OF CALCULUS TO THE TOOTH SURFACE

The following modes of attachment have been described.

1. The calculus attachment may be mediated through an organic pellicle or cuticle-like structure.
2. There is close adaptation of calculus undersurface depressions to the gently sloping mounds of the unaltered cementum surface.
3. The attachment may occur by calculus matrix penetrating into the carious defects and other surface irregularities, such as cracks and resorption lacunae and getting locked mechanically.
4. Masses of bacteria which penetrate the cementum were continuous with those in the calculus.

Calculus embedded deeply in cementum may appear morphologically similar to cementum and has been termed calculo-cementum.

88. HABIT AND PERIODONTAL DISEASE

Habit is an important factor in the initiation and progression of periodontal disease. Frequently, the presence of an unsuspected habit is revealed in patients who have failed to respond to periodontal therapy. Habits of significance may be:

  i. Neuroses—such as lip and cheek biting, tooth pick biting and wedging between the teeth, tongue thrusting, finger nail biting and bruxism.

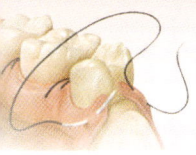

ii. Occupational habits—such as the holding of nails in the mouth as practiced by cobblers, upholsterers and carpenters.

iii. Miscellaneous habits—such as pipe or cigarette smoking, tobacco chewing, incorrect methods of tooth brushing, thumb sucking and mouth breathing.

89. TONGUE THRUSTING

Tongue thrusting entails persistent, forceful wedging of the tongue against the teeth, particularly in the anterior region. Instead of the dorsum of the tongue being placed against the palate with the tip behind the maxillary teeth during swallowing, the tongue is thrust forward against the anterior teeth (Fig. 4.34). Tongue thrusting causes excessive lateral pressure, which may be traumatic to the periodontium. It causes spreading and tilting of the anterior teeth, with an open bite anteriorly, posteriorly or in the premolar area. Tongue thrusting also results in altered inclination of teeth which in turn causes food accumulation at the gingival margin. Loss of proximal contact leads to food impaction. Tongue thrusting is an important contributing factor in pathologic tooth migration.

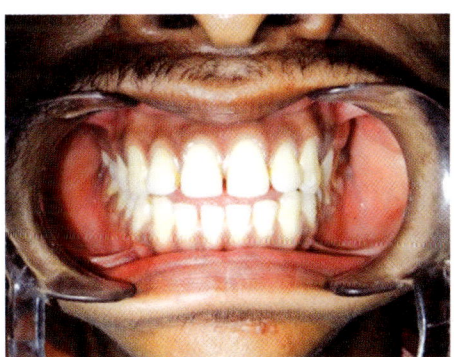

Fig. 4.34: Tongue thrusting

90. BRUXISM

Bruxism is the grinding or clenching of the teeth when the individual is not chewing or swallowing. Clenching is the

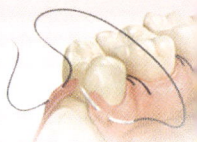

continuous or intermittent closure of the jaws under vertical pressure. Bruxism can occur as brief, rhythmic, strong contraction of the jaw muscles during eccentric lateral jaw movements or in maximum intercuspation, called clenching. Bruxism often occurs without any neurologic disorders or defects and can be viewed as a phenomenon present in healthy individuals.

Bruxism may lead to teeth wear, fractures of the teeth, muscle hypertrophy, masticatory myalgia, etc.

It is now clear that nocturnal (night time) bruxism is different from diurnal (day time) with different causes and requiring different treatment.

Most people are not aware of a bruxism, until it is brought to their attention. Wear from bruxism can be observed as facet on the tooth surface.

Bruxism can occur in any stage of sleep but is most common during the transition from deeper stage of sleep to lighter stage of sleep. It is most common in stage II (rapid eye movement— REM)

Bruxism occurring during REM sleep may be the most damaging. It is estimated that 5% of individuals brux to a pathologic extent. It is not a brain dysfunction but a CNS instability that occurs idiopathically.

Bruxism has been considered a multifactorial psychosomatic phenomenon. It has been suggested that occlusal malrelation-ships or interferences may precipitate bruxism when combined with nervous tension.

Treatment of Bruxism

1. Specific behavioral therapies.
2. If required, medications, such as diazepam.
3. The night guard appliance remains the most universal and effective long-term means of intercepting the effects of bruxism.
4. Coronoplasty plays a role in treating bruxism in connection with recently placed dental restoration.

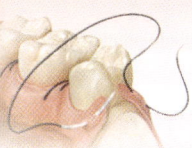

91. MOUTH BREATHING HABIT AND ITS EFFECT ON PERIODONTIUM

Gingivitis is often associated with mouth breathing. This habit may result from a number of factors.

The clinical characteristics of mouth breathing may be present in non-mouth breathers when malposed and protruding teeth prevent the normal closure of the lips (incomplete lip closure).

It has been suggested that the gingival changes result from the irritation of excessive drying. Its harmful effect is generally attributed to irritation from surface dehydration.

Gingivitis and gingival enlargement are often seen in mouth breathers. The gingiva appears red and shiny. The maxillary anterior region is the common site of such involvement. In many cases, the altered gingiva is clearly demarcated from adjacent unexposed normal gingiva. Tendency to bleed on instrumentation is increased, gingival pockets are usually present.

Treatment consists of elimination or correction of the cause of the mouth breathing. The following measures may be useful: (i) application of petroleum jelly to the gingiva before retiring, (ii) correction of sleeping position, (iii) correction of nasal obstruction, (iv) use of mouth screen during sleep, (v) plaque control, if local irritants are present.

92. EFFECTS OF TOBACCO USE ON PERIODONTIUM

Tobacco use and smoking has a detrimental effect on the progression of periodontal disease and healing after therapy.

Changes in the periodontium due to smoking and smokeless tobacco:

    i. Brownish, tar-like deposits and discoloration of tooth surface. Nicotine and cotinine are deposited on the root surface (Fig. 4.35).

   ii. Diffuse grayish discoloration and leukoplakia of gingiva may occur.

  iii. Smoker's palate (nicotinic stomatitis), prominent mucous glands with inflammation of the orifices and a diffuse

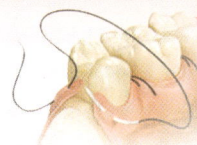

erythema or by a wrinkled, "cobblestone surface may occur".

iv. A correlation between tobacco smoking and ANUG has been clearly shown.

vi. Smoking induces an immediate transient but marked increase in gingival fluid flow, probably due to nicotine.

v. More severe gingivitis and periodontitis.

Gingivitis toxica: Characterized by destruction of gingiva and underlying bone.

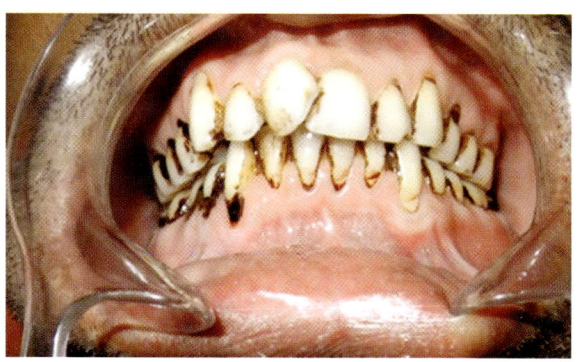

Fig. 4.35: Tobacco stains

93. SMOKING AND PERIODONTAL DISEASE

Smokers are more likely to have periodontitis than persons who had never smoked.

Effects of smoking on periodontal tissues:

1. **Microbial:** Proliferation of anaerobic fusospirochetal micro-organisms and increased colonization of periodontal pathogens in periodontal pocket is detected in smokers.

2. **Immunological:** Altered neutrophil chemotaxis, phago-cytosis and oxidative burst in smokers. Neutrophil enzymes, like collagensase, elastase and inflammatory mediators are increased in crevicular fluid in smokers.

3. **Clinical and physiological:** Greyish discoloration and hyperkeratosis of gingiva.
   • Decreased gingival blood vessels with increased inflam-mation but less severe clinical signs of inflammation

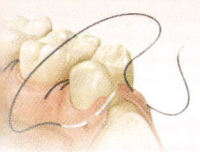

- Transient increase in GCF flow after smoking followed by decrease for prolonged period, with bleeding.
- Increased time needed to recover from local anesthesia.

Effect of smoking on response to periodontal therapy:

A. Non-surgical therapy:
- Decreased clinical response to scaling and root planing
- Decreased reduction in pocket depth
- Decreased gain in clinical attachment

B. Surgery and implants:
- Decreased pocket depth reduction and decreased gain in attachment level after flap surgery.
- Decreased bone regeneration, failure in GTR therapy, deterioration of furcation after therapy.
- Failure of osseointegration detected in some smokers.

C. Maintenance therapy: Increased pocket depth and decreased gain in attachment after surgery detected in maintenance phase, if the patient continues to smoke.

94. TOOTHBRUSH TRAUMA

Alterations in gingiva and/or tooth surface due to aggressive brushing in horizontal or rotary fashion can be acute or chronic.

  i. **Acute changes:** Scuffing of the epithelial surface with denudation of the underlying connective tissue to form a painful gingival bruise. Punctate lesions are produced by penetration of the gingiva by perpendicularly aligned bristles. Painful vesicle formation in traumatized areas is also seen. Diffuse erythema and denudation of the attached gingiva throughout the mouth may be a feature of overzealous brushing. Acute gingival abscess occurs when a tooth brush bristle gets embedded and retained in the gingiva.

 ii. **Chronic changes:** Chronic toothbrush trauma results in gingival recession with denudation of root surface. Often gingival margin is enlarged and appears to be "piled up". Linear grooves extending from marginal to the attached gingivae may be present. The gingival inflammation

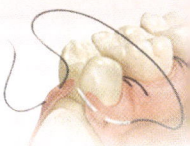

occurs due to improper use of dental floss, wooden interdental stimulators and toothpicks.

95. FACTORS FAVORING PLAQUE RETENTION

For their role in enhancing plaque retention and accumulation, the following factors are the most frequently found contributors to inflammatory gingival or periodontal disease.

Root surfaces: Coronal or radicular niches and concavities harbors plaque and cannot be reached with present day therapeutic aids.

Inadequate restorations: Restorative procedures can affect the periodontal tissues by way of faulty restorations which can cause plaque accumulation. Overhanging margins of restorations one of the most frequently found factors enhancing plaque accumulation. The restored contours, contacts and marginal ridge levels also play a role in the accumulation and retention of dentobacterial plaque.

Tooth position: Overcrowding of teeth often contributes to the accumulation of plaque and hampers its removal.

Removable partial dentures: Removable partial dentures can affect periodontal health adversely in three ways:

1. Mechanical irritation from dentures can causes gingival sloughing and even osseous destruction.
2. Dentures can cause plaque accumulation/retention where denture material approximate gingival tissues.
3. Occlusal and retentive denture designs can become traumatogenic to the attachment apparatus.

Orthodontic appliance: In and around the orthodontic bands and plate, plaque accumulation and retention is excess.

Calculus: With an increase in the specificity of experimental parameters in recent years, dentobacterial plaque and host response have replaced calculus as primary etiologic factors in inflammatory periodontal disease. However, the ability of calculus to enhance accumulation and retention of plaque cannot be overlooked.

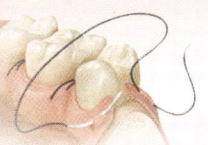

Caries: Cervical caries create conditions for continued accumulation and retention of plaque.

Periodontal pocket: The pocket becomes a reservoir for the retention of subgingival plaque and continued periodontal destruction.

Habits: Habit is an important factor for retention of plaque and progression of periodontal disease, e.g. tongue thrusting and mouth breathing.

96. CAUSES OF RECURRENCE OF PERIODONTAL DISEASE

In periodontics, the degree of success is variable. The causes for the recurrence of periodontal disease are varied and they could be grouped as:

A. Lack of cooperation by the patient

B. The therapeutic judgment of the operator

C. Knowledge concerning the intrinsic factors in the cause of periodontal disease.

The causes of recurrence are:

1. Improper diagnosis and incomplete treatment
2. Incomplete scaling and root planing in the maintenance program.
3. Inappropriate or improper dental restorations or prosthesis.
4. Intrinsic or other factors beyond your or the patients control (e.g. diabetes, or compromised immune responses)
5. Inadequate oral hygiene by the patient.

Recurrent periodontal disease is characterized by one or all of the following symptoms:

1. Sulci that bleed when probed
2. Increased pocket depth
3. Continued bone loss
4. Increased mobility of the tooth/teeth.
5. Pus discharge on palpation at the gingival margin

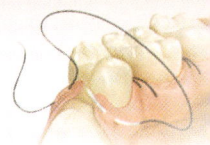

97. GINGIVAL CHANGES ASSOCIATED WITH PREGNANCY

Pregnancy gingivitis: The severity of gingivitis is increased in pregnancy. At the same time, pregnancy itself does not cause gingivitis. Pregnancy accentuates the gingival response to plaque and modifies the resultant clinical picture. Pronounced ease of bleeding is the most striking clinical feature. The color of the gingiva varies from bright red to a bluish red described as "old rose". The marginal and papillary gingiva is edematous, smooth and shiny, the appearance, sometimes, is raspberry-like. The gingival changes are usually painless unless complicated by acute infection.

Pregnancy tumor: In some cases, the inflamed gingiva forms discrete "tumor" like masses, referred to as "pregnancy tumors". It usually appears during second or third month of pregnancy.

The pregnancy tumor appears as a discrete, mushroom-like flattened spherical mass that protrudes from the gingival margin or, more frequently from the interproximal space and attached by a sessile or pedunculated at base. Generally dusky red or magenta, it has a smooth, glistening surface that frequently exhibits numerous deep red, pinpoint markings. It is superficial lesion usually of semi-firm consistency. It is usually painless, its size and shape foster accumulation of debris under its margin and interfere with occlusion, in which case painful ulceration may occur.

Microbiology: The microorganisms whose proportion increase significantly during pregnancy are *Prevotella intermedia and Bacteroides melaninogenicus.*

Course of the disease: The severity of gingivitis is increased during pregnancy beginning in the second or third month and becomes more severe by the eighth month and decreases during the ninth. Plaque accumulation follows a similar pattern. The correlation between gingivitis and the quantity of plaque is greater after parturition than during pregnancy, which suggests that pregnancy introduces other factors that aggravate the gingival response to local irritants.

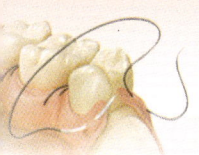

Also tooth mobility, pocket depth and gingival fluid are increased in pregnancy.

98. ORAL CONTRACEPTIVES AND GINGIVAL CHANGES

Oral contraceptives alter the circulatory levels of estrogen and progesterone and thereby aggravate the gingival response to local irritants in manner similar to that of pregnancy, and when taken for a period more than one and half year, increases periodontal destruction. The response produces a gingivitis that is usually not as severe but does resemble gingivitis during pregnancy. The change in color from pink to red and the interdental and marginal gingival consistency from firm to edematous, smooth and shiny is characteristic feature in this type.

99. MENOPAUSAL GINGIVOSTOMATITIS (SENILE ATROPHIC GINGIVITIS)

It is one of the uncommon conditions. This condition occurs during the menopause or in post-menopausal period. In this condition, the gingiva and the oral mucosa is dry and shiny, the color varies from paleness to redness which bleeds easily. There is fissuring in the mucobuccal fold in some cases. At times the patient complains of a dry, burning sensation throughout the oral cavity, associated with extreme sensitivity to thermal changes and abnormal taste sensation described as "salty", "peppery" or sour. Sometimes bone loss is also evident. There is difficulty with removable partial prostheses. The signs and symptoms of menopausal gingivostomatitis are comparable with those of chronic desquamative gingivitis to some extent.

100. DIABETES AND PERIODONTAL DISEASE

Diabetes mellitus includes disturbed glucose utilization because of the pathologic condition in the beta cells of the pancreas. Diabetes leads to protein breakdown, degenerative processes, lowered resistance to infection, vascular changes and an

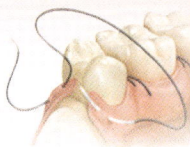

increase in the severity of the inflammatory reactions. Phagocytosis is impaired in hyperglycemia and ketoacidosis. Chemotaxis of PMN leukocytes is impaired in the absence of insulin.

Clinical Features

- Tendency towards abscess formation
- Diabetic periodontoclasia
- Enlarged gingiva, sessile or pedunculated gingival polyps
- Bone loss
- Increased mobility of teeth
- Delayed postsurgical healing

Treatment

If signs of diabetes are noticed in a patient, further investigations via laboratory studies and history taking should be performed, because periodontal treatment in the patient with uncontrolled diabetes is contraindicated. After consultation with the patient's physician, following guidelines should be followed in treatment of diabetics.

1. Prophylactic antibiotics
2. Morning appointments after breakfast are ideal because of optimal insulin levels.
3. Handling of tissues as atraumatically and as minimally (less than 2 hours) as possible.
4. Diet recommendations to maintain a proper glucose balance.
5. Frequent recall appointment and fastidious home oral care.

101. STRESS AND PERIODONTAL DISEASE

Psychological conditions, particularly stress have been implicated as risk indicators for periodontal disease. The most notable example is the relationship between stress and acute necrotizing ulcerative gingivitis (ANUG). The presence of ANUG in soldiers stressed by wartime conditions in the

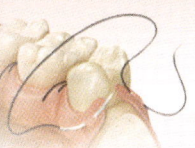

trenches led to one of the early diagnostic term namely "trench mouth". The association between stress and chronic periodontitis is elusive. However, the relationship between stress and smoking in the aggressive periodontitis has been shown to some extent. Increasing evidence suggests that emotional stress also may influence the extent and severity of chronic periodontitis. Stress and depression may also influence the outcome of periodontal therapy.

102. GENERAL ADAPTATION SYNDROME (SELYE)

Stress, such as trauma, muscular fatigue, drug intoxication and nervous stimuli affect the body and produce interrelated, nonspecific changes in the tissues. As described by Selye, the composite of the systemic reactions that result from continued exposure to stress is termed the general adaptation syndrome (GAS). The general adaptation syndrome is generalized group of physiologic mechanisms that represent an attempt by the body to resist the damaging effect of stress. The general adaptation syndrome develops in three stages:

1. The initial response—"The alarm reaction"
2. The adaptation to stress—"The resistance stage"
3. A final stage marked by inability to maintain adaptation to the stress—"The exhaustion stage".

In the alarm reaction, no significant changes are seen. In the late stages, osteoporosis of alveolar bone, epithelial sloughing, degeneration of the periodontal ligament, and reduced osteoblastic activity are noted in chronic stress situations. Stress also leads to delayed healing of the connective tissue and bone in experimental animals.

103. NUTRITIONAL CONSIDERATION IN PERIODONTICS

The mouth mirrors good health, so the determination of the quality and quantity of nutrients appropriate for good health can be added by observing the effects of particular nutrients on the oral tissues.

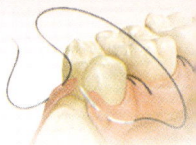

Nutrition may influence the growth, development and metabolic activities of the periodontium. Response of the periodontium to the plaque bacteria is affected by its innate resistance to infection which depends on the nutritional status of the individual.

Nutritional deficiency may not initiate periodontal disease but perpetuates it. Therefore in the treatment, nutritional counseling to improve the systemic resistance should be considered along with the conventional periodontal treatment.

Thus adequate nutrition is essential. Diet adequate in calories, proteins, vitamins and minerals must be instituted. At the same time the physical character of the diet is important. Firm, fibrous foods benefit the gingiva by giving the cleansing action and mechanical stimulation, thereby minimizing the accumulation of microbial plaque and irritating food debris. It also provides functional stimulation for maintenance of periodontal ligament and alveolar bone.

Most of the deficiencies of the vitamins reflect in the oral cavity. Vitamin A deficiency results in keratinizing metaplasia of epithelium and increased susceptibility to infection. B-complex deficiency leads to gingivitis, cheilosis, glossitis, etc. while vitamin C deficiency results in scurvy. Vitamin D and calcium deficiency can cause defects in formation and calcification of bones.

104. HISTOLOGIC AND CLINICAL PICTURE, AND TREATMENT OF SCORBUTIC GINGIVITIS (SCURVY)

Scurvy, i.e. vitamin C deficiency is characterized by hemorrhagic diathesis and retardation of wound healing.

Vitamin C and periodontal disease:

1. Vitamin C deficiency influences the metabolism of collagen, thereby affecting the ability of the tissues of the periodontium to regenerate.

2. Vitamin C deficiency interferes with bone formation, leading to loss of periodontal bone.

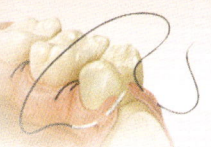

3. Vitamin C deficiency increases the permeability of the oral mucosa to endotoxins and insulin and of normal human crevicular epithelium to dextran.

4. Vitamin C deficiency may affect chemotactic and migratory action of leukocytes, without influencing their phagocytic activity.

5. Integrity of the microvasculature of the periodontium is affected, along with vascular response to bacterial irritation and wound healing.

6. Vitamin C deficiency may interfere with the ecologic equilibrium of bacteria in plaque.

Characteristic Features

1. Increased susceptibility to infection

2. Impaired wound healing

3. Bleeding, swollen gingiva

4. Loosened teeth

5. Gingivitis with enlargement hemorrhagic, bluish red gingiva.

The gingival consistency is soft and friable with smooth and shiny surface. Vitamin C deficiency does not cause periodontal pockets; local bacterial factors are required for pocket formation to occur.

Vitamin C is abundant in fruits and vegetables, the daily requirement (dietary) of vitamin C which is the recommended intake for normal persons is 30 mg/day.

105. PROTEIN DEFICIENCY AND PERIODONTIUM

Protein calorie malnutrition is a common problem in developing countries. It promotes the development of acute periodontal lesions in children. In contrast, a relative deficiency in calcium compared to phosphorus in the diet may play a role in the development of periodontal disease in adults.

Protein calorie malnutrition (kwashiorkor) is by far the most widespread nutritional disorders. Protein depletion

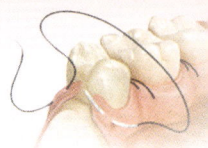

results in hypoproteinemia with many pathologic changes, such as decreased resistance to infection, slow wound healing. Lesions of the buccal mucosa may be observed along with significant generalized osteoporosis and alveolar bone loss.

Protein deficiency accentuates the destructive effects of local irritants and occlusal trauma upon the periodontal tissues, but the initiation of gingival inflammation and its severity depends upon the local irritants. Hence, protein deficiency affects the connective tissue fibers in the gingiva and periodontal ligament, pronounced osteoporosis of the alveolar bone and marked retardation in deposition of cementum.

Some of the changes seen in the periodontium of experimental animals due to protein deficiency:

1. Degeneration of connective tissue of gingiva and periodontal ligament
2. Osteoporosis of alveolar bone
3. Retardation in the cementum deposition
4. Delayed wound healing

106. PERIODONTAL MEDICINE

It is a rapidly emerging branch of periodontology based on evidences establishing a strong relationship between periodontal and systemic condition.

Systemic disease reflecting in oral cavity is well-known. But now studies suggest the periodontal infection as a risk factor for some of the systemic diseases or conditions such as:

- Cardiovascular disease (AMI)
- Diabetes mellitus
- Stroke
- Premature delivery or low-birth weight (LBW)
- Respiratory disease (COPD)
- Rheumatoid arthritis

1. Cardiovascular disease/AMI; stroke and respiratory disease

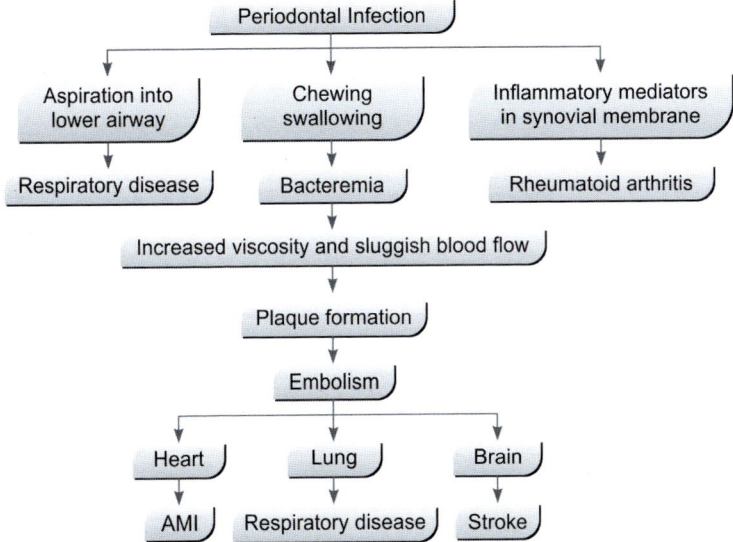

2. Diabetes

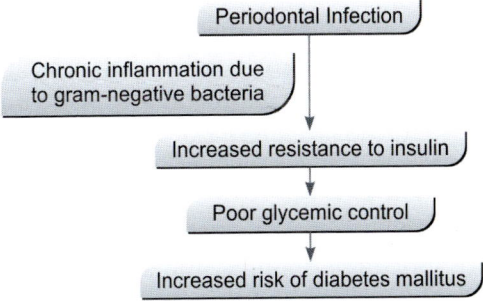

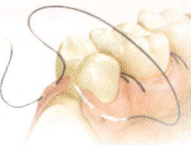

3. Premature delivery or preterm low birth weight.

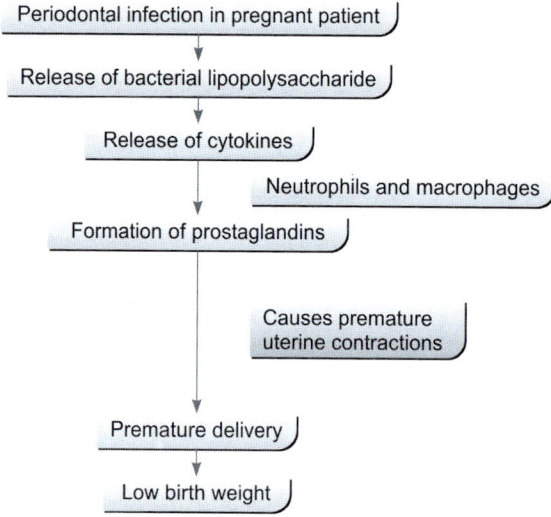

107. HALITOSIS/ORAL MALODOR/BAD BREATH

Halitosis may arise from odors that are emitted from the oral cavity, nasal passages, sinuses, pharynx, and lungs.

Intraoral causes: Poor oral hygiene which allows food debris to stagnate and dental plaque to accumulate around teeth is probably the most important factor in causing halitosis. Other factors include putrifaction of saliva, dental caries, coated tongue, periodontal disease, dehydration states, oral infections and smoking.

Oral infections are accompanied by a fetid breath, ANUG, Noma, causes offensive characteristics odor.

Dehydration of oral tissues, for any reason causes a fetid breath, because it leads to a reduced salivary flow and hence less cleansing action.

Periodontitis, gingivitis, and caries, artificial dentures, smokers, healing surgical or extraction wounds are associated with mouth odors. Periodontitis causes the greatest odor.

The use of tobacco and smoking gives characteristics odor in the mouth. Smoker's breath is very pungent.

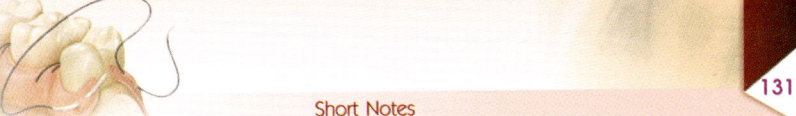
Also periodontal pockets and surgery associated with bleeding and necrosis, gives odor.

There are numerous causes of halitosis but there can be little doubt the microbial plaque is a primary etiological factor. Volatile sulfide compounds (VSCs), such as hydrogen sulfide or methyl mercaptan produced by gram-negative, anaerobic bacteria are responsible for oral malodor. Tissue destruction and putrefaction of amino acids by bacteria leads to production of VSCs. Therefore, malodor intensity is much greater in the presence of periodontal disease. Hence, early plaque control will not only prevent periodontal disease but also greatly reduce halitosis of local origin.

Extraoral causes: Diseases, such as pharyngitis, postnasal drip lung abscesses and malignant tumors, give foul odor.

Diagnosis of oral malodor can be made by medical history and clinical and laboratory investigations. Sometimes organoleptic devices, such as halimeter can also be used. Treatment of halitosis is based on elimination of etiological factors.

108. DIAGNOSTIC AIDS IN PERIODONTICS

Proper diagnosis is essential for intelligent treatment. Periodontal diagnosis consists of analysis of the case and an evaluation of the clinical signs and symptoms, as well as the results of the various tests and the diagnostic aids to identify the patient's problem.

Diagnostic Aids

1. Case History

A. **Medical history:**
   a. For diagnosis of oral manifestations of systemic diseases.
   b. For detection of systemic conditions affecting perio-dontium and/or requiring special modifications while treatment.

B. **Dental history:**
   a. To explore the source of the patients chief complaint.
   b. To determine whether emergency treatment is required.

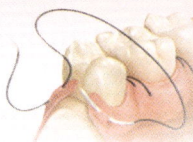

2. Clinical Photograph

Color photographs are useful for recording the appearance of the tissues before and after the treatment.

3. Casts

Casts from dental impressions are extremely useful adjuncts in the oral examination. Casts provide a view of lingual cuspal relationships. They indicate:

   i. The position of gingival margins

   ii. The position and inclination of teeth

  iii. Proximal contact relationships

  iv. Food impaction areas

   v. They serve as visual aids in discussion with the patient

  vi. Are useful for pretreatment and post-treatment comparisons, as well as for reference at check-up visits. They are important records of the dentition before it is altered by the treatment.

4. Hemogram

Complete hemogram which includes blood cell counts and differential leulocyte count, bleeding and clotting time, hemoglobin assay and erythrocyte sedimentation rate are essential blood screening tests.

5. Microbiological Diagnostic Aids

1. Dark field/phase contrast microscopy

2. Culture methods

3. Immunological assays

4. Immunofluorescence—direct/indirect

5. Latex agglutination

6. Flow cytometry

7. Enzyme-linked immunosorbent assay (ELISA)

8. Enzymatic methods, ex. BANA.

9. DNA probes.

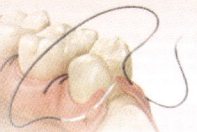

6. Radiographic Survey

a. Intraoral radiographs provide an overall picture of the distribution and severity of bone destruction in periodontal disease.

b. Panoramic radiographs are simple and convenient method of obtaining a survey view of the dental arch and surrounding structures. They are helpful for the detection of developmental anomalies, pathologic lesions of the teeth and jaws and fractures, and for dental screening examinations of large groups (Fig. 4.36).

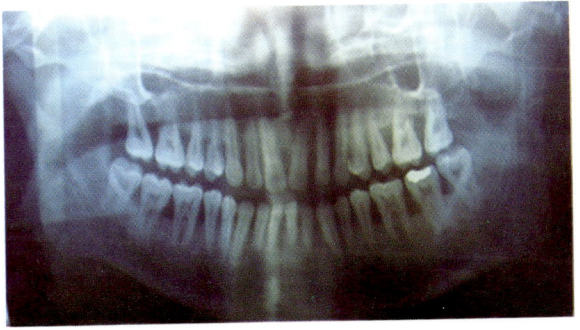

Fig. 4.36: Panoramic radiograph showing aggressive periodontitis

7. Advanced Diagnostic Aids

1. Xeroradiography is process by which X-ray images are recorded by means of xerographic copying method. It offers the advantage of an "edge enhancement" effect that may permit better visualization of crestal bone height and to some extent soft tissues surrounding the teeth.

2. Absorptiometry.

3. Photodensitometric analysis

4. Subtraction radiography

5. Computer assisted densitometric image analysis (CADIA).

6. CBCT

8. Biochemical Diagnosis

These include tests based on host-derived factors like, saliva,

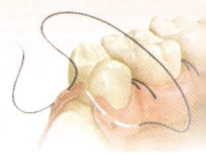

serum, GCF, urine, blood cells, e.g. 40 components of GCF have been studied under three main groups:

a. Host-derived enzymes
b. Tissue breakdown products
c. Inflammatory mediators

9. Laboratory Aids in Diagnosis

a. **Biopsy:** The diagnosis of neoplasms should be established by microscopic examination.

b. **Exfoliative cytology:** It is a diagnostic procedure consisting of the microscopic examination of cells obtained by scraping the surface of the suspected area or by rinsing the oral cavity.

c. **Smears:** Material from lesions may be obtained and submitted to the laboratory for confirmation of diagnosis of acute gingival conditions.

109. BANA

(Full form: N–Benzoyl–DL–arginine–2–naphthylamide) Enzymatic profile of plaque bacteria can be used to detect the presence of periodontal pathogens in subgingival plaque samples. Various enzyme diagnostic kits have been developed for the identification of pure cultures of plaque isolates.

These enzyme assays are helpful in identification of important periodontal pathogens, such as *P. gingivalis,* because most of these demonstrate positive trypsin-like reaction. The activity of this enzyme is measured with the hydrolysis of the colorless substrate N–benzoyl–DL–arginine–2–naphthylamide (BANA). When hydrolysis takes place, it releases the chromophoro β-naphthylamide which changes to orange red when a drop of fast garnet is added to solution.

Diagnostic kits (Perioscan) have been developed using this reaction for identification of bacteria in plaque.

It is seen that shallow pockets exhibited only 10% positive BANA reactions as compared to deep pockets (80–90%).

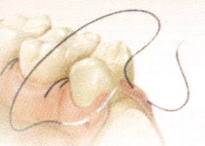

110. PERIOTRON

Measurement of flow of gingival crevicular fluid can be used to detect degree of gingival inflammation in initial stages. An electronic device Periotron is used to measure gingival crevicular fluid flow.

Method

1. Gingival crevicular fluid is collected by placing the filter paper strips (Periopaper) at the entrance of the crevice.
2. These wetted strips then inserted into the slot present in periotron device.
3. Periotron measures the change in capacitance across the wetted strips and convert it to a digital readout.

The measurements achieved by periotron, were the easiest and quickest, showing high correlation with other clinical gingival indices. However, the results can be affected by room temperature, humidity and placement of filter paper strips.

111. RADIOGRAPHS IN PERIODONTAL DIAGNOSIS

The radiograph is a valuable aid in the diagnosis of periodontal disease, the determination of prognosis, and the evaluation of the outcome of treatment. It is, however, an adjunct to the clinical examination, not a substitute for it. Radiographs have a two-dimensional representation of three-dimensional structures. The radiographic image tends to show less severe bone loss than is actually present (Figs 4.37A and B). Radiographs can give some of the following information:

1. **Interdental bone height and presence of a lamina dura:** Because of the facial and lingual bony plates are obscured by the relatively dense root structure, radiographic evaluation of bone changes in periodontal disease is based mainly on the appearance of the interdental septum.

   The interdental septum presents a thin, radiopaque border adjacent to the periodontal ligament and at the crest referred to as lamina dura. It appears as a continuous white line. Lamina dura represents the bone surface lining the tooth socket.

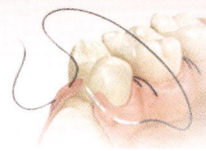

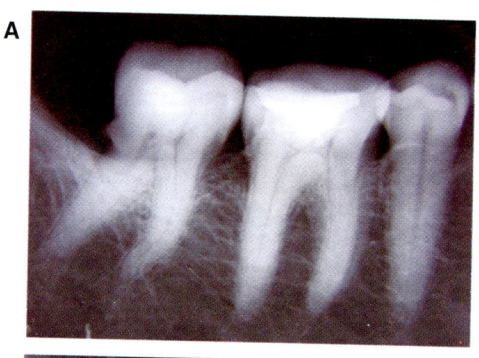

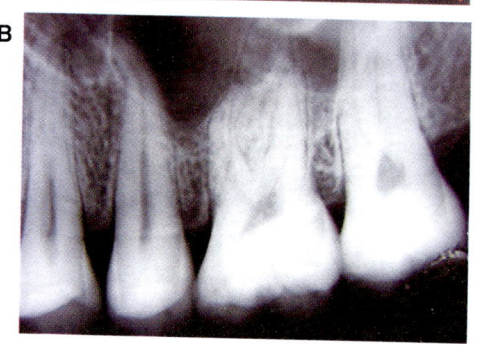

Fig. 4.37: (A) Ideal IOPA mandibular; (B) Ideal IOPA maxillary

2. **Trabecular patterns:** The loss of trabeculations caused by disuse atrophy will be readily apparent around teeth long out of occlusion and around extraction sites.

3. **Areas of bone destruction:** The amount, distribution and pattern of bone destruction can be confirmed along with clinical probing. Bone loss in furcations and its periapical involvement can be judged.

4. **Width of periodontal ligament space:** Radiograph is a valuable aid in understanding the periodontal ligament space.

5. **Crown-to-root ratio:** This can be estimated by radiograph. Besides this, radiograph can evaluate, the size, shape, and form of the crown as it relates to the size, shape, form, number and position of roots, and quality as well as quantity of the remaining bone and attachment.

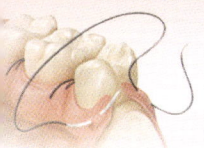
6. **Amount of bone loss:** In periodontal disease, radiograph is an indirect method for determining the amount of bone loss in disease. It shows the amount of bone remaining rather than the bone lost. Amount of bone lost is estimated to be the difference between the physiologic bone level and the height of remaining bone.

7. **Distribution of bone loss:** It indicates the location of destructive local factor in different areas of the mouth and in relation to different surfaces of the same tooth.

8. **Patterns of bone destruction:**

   • *Horizontal bone loss:* Reduction in height with the crest horizontal to long axis of adjacent teeth.

   • *Vertical bone loss:* Reduction in height with the crest perpendicular to long axis of the adjacent teeth.

   Radiographs can also be used to detect interdental craters, furcation involvement, aggressive periodontitis, trauma from occlusion and abscess.

112. GINGIVAL BIOPSY

It is important in the diagnosis of some gingival disturbances, particularly, if neoplastic lesions are present. Microscopic study of gingival biopsy specimens is sometimes the only method of detecting local and systemic interrelationships that cannot be discerned by clinical examination.

It is one of the laboratory aids in diagnosis. The diagnosis of neoplasms, and differentiating the varied lesions, such as different types of gingival enlargements, desquamative gingivitis, benign mucous membrane pemphigoids, pemphigus, and herpetic gingivostomatitis are suspected.

There are several biopsy techniques, such as incisional biopsy, punch biopsy and curettage.

The tissue should not be crushed or mutilated. It should be placed in fixative, immediately. 10% formalin is an acceptable fixative.

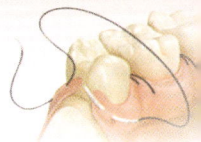

Exfoliative cytology: It is diagnostic procedure consisting of the microscopic examination of cells obtained by scraping the surface of the suspected area or by rinsing the oral cavity. Exfoliative cytology is not a substitute for biopsy, but it is valuable if a biopsy cannot be done for some reason and also if large group of people are to be screened for the malignancy.

113. GINGIVAL RECESSION

Recession is the exposure of the root surface by an apical shift in the position of the gingiva. There are two types of recession, (i) visible, which is clinically observable and (ii) hidden, which is covered by gingiva and can only be measured by inserting a probe to the level of epithelial attachment. Recession refers to the location of the marginal gingiva not its conditions. Receded gingiva is often inflamed but may be normal except for its position. Recession may be localized to a tooth or a group of teeth or may be generalized throughout the mouth. The cause of gingival recession, whether localized or generalized, is not always easy to determine. The following factors may be considered:

Physiologic: Related to aging.

Pathologic

1. Tooth brush injury
2. Ortho treatment sometimes results in recession if the bony plate is thin.
3. Periodontal traumatism
4. Inflammatory periodontal disease
5. Faulty tooth alignment
6. Anatomic abnormalities such as dehiscence.
7. Deleterious habits (pressure of foreign objects, finger nails, etc.)
8. Friction from soft tissues (gingival ablation).
9. Surgical treatment of inflammatory periodontal disease.
10. High frenal attachment.
11. Pressure from mastication.

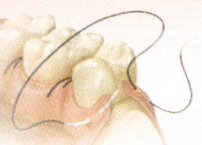

Susceptibility to recession is influenced by:
a. Position of tooth in the arch,
b. Root bone angle, and
c. Mesiodistal curvature of the tooth surface.

Classification of Gingival Recession (by Miller)

Class I: Marginal tissue does not extend to the mucogingival junction with no interdental bone or soft tissue loss. (narrow or wide)

Class II: Recession extending beyond mucogingival junction with no interdental bone or soft tissue loss. (wide and narrow)

Class III: Recession extending beyond mucogingival junction with bone and soft tissue loss interdentally.

Class IV: Recession extending beyond the mucogingival junction with severe bone and soft tissue loss interdentally

Clinical Significance

Exposed root surfaces are susceptible to caries. Wearing away of the cementum exposed by recession leaves an underlying dentinal surface that is extremely sensitive, particularly to touch.

Hyperemia of the pulp and associated symptoms may also result from exposure of the root surface. Interproximal recession creates spaces in which plaque, food, and bacteria can accumulate.

114. ROOT HYPERSENSITIVITY AS PERIODONTAL PROBLEM

Root surfaces exposed by gingival recession may be hypersensitive to thermal or tactile stimulation. The hypersensitivity is most often related to a transient pulpal hyperemia resulting from the scaling and root planing or the removal or shrinkage of gingival tissues that provide a protective covering for the roots. If the microorganisms are allowed to accumulate regularly on the freshly scaled open dentinal tubules, the nerve endings will be continually irritated and sensitive.

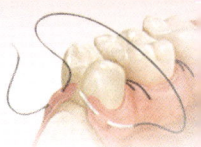

The following precautions are helpful in the prevention of tooth hypersensitivity.

1. Proper plaque control before and after periodontal surgery.

2. Application of periodontal dressing on the treated teeth until the gingival tissues healed sufficiently to allow tooth brushing.

3. Temporary restorations for carious lesions before the periodontal surgery.

The treatment of hypersensitivity should always begin by perfecting plaque control and sufficient time for pulp to adjust the root instrumentation and the increased root exposure. However, if the tooth sensitivity persists, several office and home treatments are available.

1. Burnishing with a sodium fluoride paste into the sensitive area on the root.

2. Daily rinsing with a 0.5% stannous fluoride solution.

3. Office and home application of a commercial desensitizing preparations. In office, iontophoresis can also be used with varnishes, dentin bonding agents and LASER.

4. Regular use of desensitizing tooth paste, tooth powders, etc.

These procedures are also useful and effective in the treatment of tooth sensitivity associated with idiopathic tooth erosion and gingival recession.

115. TOOTH MOBILITY

All teeth have a slight degree of physiologic mobility, which varies for different teeth and at different times of the day. Mobility beyond the physiologic range is termed abnormal or pathologic. Mobility is graded clinically by holding the tooth firmly between the handles of two metallic instruments or with one metallic instrument and one finger and moved in all directions (Fig. 4.38). Mobilometers or periodontometers are mechanical or electronic devices for the precise measurement of tooth mobility.

It occurs in two stages:

1. **Intial or intrasocket stage:** In this, tooth moves within the confines of the periodontal ligament.

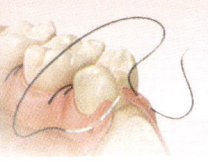

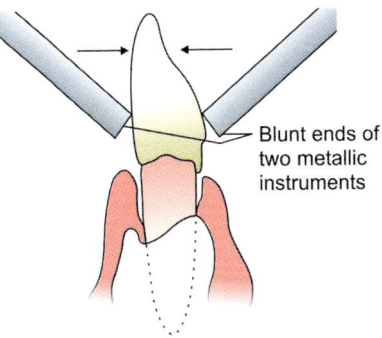

Blunt ends of
two metallic
instruments

Fig. 4.38: Evaluation of mobility

2. Secondary stage: It occurs gradually and includes elastic deformation of the alveolar bone in response to increased horizontal forces.

Mobility is graded according to the ease and extent of tooth movement.

Grade 0: Physiologic or normal mobility.

Grade I: Slightly more than normal or movement of tooth in both the facial and the lingual directions but less than 1 mm range.

Grade II: Moderately more than normal or movement of tooth in faciolingual and mesiodistal directions and more than 1 mm range.

Grade III: Severe mobility faciolingually and/or mesiodistally combined with vertical displacement or movement of tooth in all the directions with ease and more than 1 mm with easy depression. For practical purposes, grade three mobile teeth are functionless.

Tooth mobility is evaluated in a periodontal examination because it is one of the signs of periodontal disease that can indicate the extent of periodontal destruction and affect the outcome of successful treatment. In general, increased tooth mobility is related to one or more of the following pathologic conditions: (i) Loss of tooth support due to bone loss causes tooth mobility, (ii) trauma from occlusion—injury produced

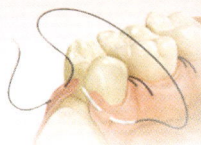

by excessive occlusal forces or increased forces because of high filling, abnormal occlusal habits are common causes of tooth mobility, (iii) extension of inflammation from the gingiva or from the periapical area into the periodontal ligament, (iv) the acute periapical abscess may increase tooth mobility, (v) tooth mobility is increased in pregnancy and is sometimes associated with hormonal imbalance.

The prognosis for successfully treating teeth with increased mobility varies, depending on the reasons for the mobility, and the degree of control the therapist has over the causative factors.

116. PERIODONTAL SPLINTS

Periodontal disease impairs tooth support and permits secondary traumatism to occur. As a result, teeth may loosen, and the alveolar bone may be subjected to additional damage. Thus reduction of tooth mobility is an important objective of periodontal therapy. Mobile teeth can be splinted to improve healing.

Definition: Splint is an appliance for immobilization or stabilization of injured or diseased parts and/or mobile teeth.

It is imperative that occlusal stability and control of excessive occlusal forces be obtained first, before splinting is applied. Frequently, the modification of occlusal forces eliminates the need for a splint, as the teeth become less mobile or more stable in their position.

Occlusal forces applied to splints are shared by all teeth within the splint even if force is applied to only one section of the splint. If one tooth in a splint is in traumatic occlusal relationship, the periodontal tissues of the remaining teeth may also get injured.

Requirements of ideal splint: It should be (1) simple, (2) economic, (3) stable and efficient, (4) hygienic, (5) non-irritating, (6) esthetically acceptable, (7) it should not interfere with treatment (periodontal), (8) it should not provoke iatrogenic disease, (9) it should not interfere with phonetics, (10) it should allow oral physiotherapy techniques and, (11) it should not subject the teeth to torsional stress.

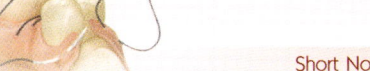

Indications for Splint

1. When moderate to advanced tooth mobility is present and cannot be treated by any other means.
2. Prior or during periodontal surgery on mobile teeth (provisional splint)
3. Permanent splints utilizing cast restorations may be placed as part of the restorative phase of therapy.

Classification of Splints

- Splints can be fixed, removable, combination of both.
- It may be temporary, provisional, permanent.
- It may be internal, external.
  The types of provisional stabilization are as follows:
  a. The reinforced resin splint for posterior teeth.
  b. Simple lingual coverage splint

Fixed Splints

a. Goal post (staplet) splint.   c. Continuous intracoronal bar.
b. The A splint   d. Endodontic splints.

Splinting Results

1. Rest is created for supporting tissues permitting repair.
2. Mobility is reduced immediately.
3. Forces are distributed to number of teeth.
4. Proximal contacts are stabilized and food impaction is prevented.
5. Migration and over eruption is prevented.
6. Masticatory function may be improved.
7. Pain and discomfort is eliminated.

117. WASTING DISEASE OF THE TEETH

Any loss of tooth substance, which is non-carious in nature and leads to formation of smooth and polished surface, is called wasting disease of the teeth. The important wasting diseases are: erosion, abrasion and attrition.

Erosion (corrosion): Sharply defined wedge shaped depression (cuneiform defect) in the cervical area of the facial tooth surface

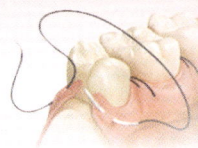

may be attributed to decalcification by acidic beverages, citrus food and/or acidic type of saliva. It usually involves enamel and sometimes dentin and cementum.

Abrasion: Saucer-shaped indentations produced by mechanical wear other than mastication. It usually starts around the cementoenamel junction and may later involve enamel or dentin.

Attrition: Occlusal or incisal wear (facet formation) resulting from functional contacts with antagonist teeth. Horizontal facets direct the forces on the long axis of the tooth which can be very well tolerated by the periodontium. However, angular facets direct forces laterally causing increased risk of periodontal destruction.

Abfraction: Occlusal overloading sometimes causes tooth flexure and mechanical microfracture and loss of tooth substance in cervical area is termed as abfraction.

118. PROGNOSIS

Definition: The prognosis is a prediction of the duration, course and termination of the disease and of its response to treatment.

The prognosis for patients with gingival disease depends on inflammation. If inflammation is the only pathologic change, the prognosis is favorable, if inflammation is associated with systemic cause or changes with hormonal disorders gingival health may be improved temporarily, but long-term prognosis depends on the control of systemic factors.

The prognosis for patients with periodontitis is:
a. Overall prognosis
b. Prognosis for individual teeth.

Overall Prognosis

It depends upon following factors:
1. Type of periodontitis
2. Assessment of bone response.
3. Application of bone factor concept—positive and negative bone factor. If the local irritants commensurate with the bone loss; the bone factor will be positive and will have better prognosis

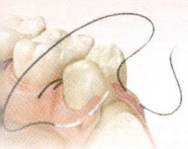

4. Height of remaining bone.
5. Patient's age.
6. Patient's systemic background.
7. Patient's attitude and desire to maintain the natural teeth.
8. Smoking.
9. Malocclusion
10. Patient's ability to maintain the oral hygiene.

Individual Tooth Prognosis

It is determined by factors, such as:
1. Mobility
2. Periodontal pocket
3. Teeth adjacent to edentulous area and the relation to adjacent teeth
4. Location of remaining bone in relation to individual tooth surface
5. Mucogingival problem
6. Infrabony pockets
7. Furcation involvement
8. Caries, nonvital teeth and root resorption
9. Tooth anomalies

119. TREATMENT PLAN

After the diagnosis and prognosis are established, treatment is planned. The treatment plan is the blueprint for the case management. It includes all procedures required for the establishment and maintenance of oral health. Periodontal treatment requires long range planning. The value of periodontal treatment to the patient is measured in year of healthful service of the entire dentition, not by the number of teeth retained at the time of treatment. A treatment plan should be developed to achieve following. Except for emergencies, no treatment should be started until the treatment plan has been established.

Treatment plan consists of following phases:

Preliminary or emergency phase: Treatment of emergencies—dental or periapical, extraction of hopeless teeth, etc.

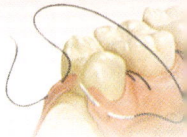

Phase I therapy (non-surgical phase): Plaque control, diet control, removal of calculus and root planing, correction of restorative and prosthetic irritational factors, local or systemic antimicrobial therapy, occlusal therapy, provisional splinting, minor orthodontic movement.

Evaluation of response to phase **I:** Rechecking pocket depth gingival inflammation, plaque, calculus, etc.

Phase II therapy (surgical phase): Periodontal surgery, including implant placement, root canal therapy.

Phase III therapy (restorative phase): Final restorations, fixed and removable prosthesis. Definitive occlusal adjustment and permanent splinting when indicated.

Phase IV therapy (maintenance phase): Instructions in oral physiotherapy, periodic recall visits, checking plaque, calculus, gingival and periodontal conditions.

Aims of Treatment Plan

Aim of treatment plan is total treatment, i.e. co-ordination of all treatment procedures for the purpose of creating a well-functioning dentition in a healthy periodontal environment.

Explaining the treatment plan to the patient involves the following steps:

a. Specificity, i.e. explaining exactly what the condition is, how it is treated and the future of treatment.

b. Starting the discussion on a positive note: Emphasizing on retention of teeth as far as possible.

c. Presenting the entire treatment plan as a unit without creating an impression that the treatment plan consists of separate procedures.

Thus the objective of every treatment plan should be welfare of the dentition as a whole.

120. RATIONALE FOR PERIODONTAL TREATMENT

Periodontal therapy should accomplish:
Local factors:
• Removal of local irritants.
• Elimination of abnormal occlusal forces.

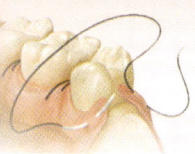

Systemic factors:
- Employed as an adjunct to local therapy
- Controlling specific complications, from acute infection or chemotherapy
- Preventing harmful effects of post-treatment bacteremia
- Host modulation

Factors Affecting Healing

Local factors:
- Resistant microorganisms.
- Excessive tissue manipulation during treatment.
- Trauma to the tissues
- Presence of foreign bodies.
- Repetitive treatment procedures that disrupt the orderly cellular activity in the healing process.

Systemic factors:
- Ageing
- Patients with generalized infections.
- Diabetic patients
- Insufficient food intake
- Hormonal imbalance.

121. NEW ATTACHMENT, REATTACHMENT AND EPITHELIAL ADAPTATION

During healing of periodontal pocket, the area is invaded by cells from oral epithelium, connective tissue, bone and periodontal ligament. When cells from periodontal ligament proliferate coronally, there is formation of cemetum and periodontal ligament (Fig. 4.39).

New attachment is the embedding of new periodontal ligament fibers into newly formed cementum and attachment of gingival epithelium to a tooth surface previously denuded by the disease. The important part in this definition is "tooth surface previously denuded by the disease." New attachment differs from reattachment. Reattachment refers to repair in areas of the root not previously exposed to the pocket such as after surgical

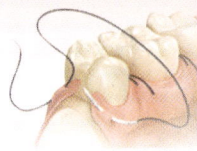

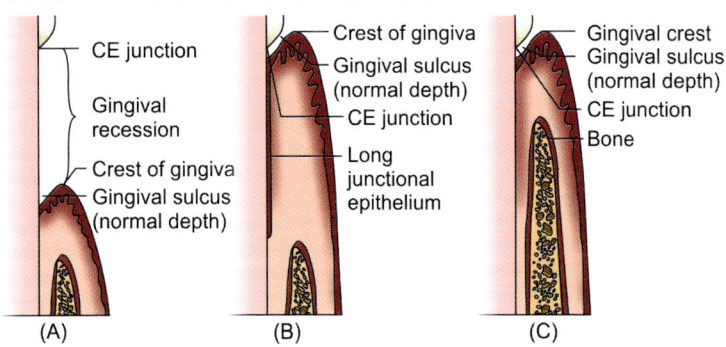

Fig. 4.39: Periodontal healing: (A) Repair by means of gingival recession; (b) Repair by means of long junctional epithelium (c) New attachment

detachment of the tissues or following traumatic tears in the cementum. Tooth fractures or the treatment of periapical lesions.

Epithelial adaptation also differs from new attachment in that it is the close apposition of the gingival epithelium to the tooth surface with no gain in height of gingival fiber attachment. The pocket is not completely obliterated although it may not permit passage of a probe.

In short, New attachment occurs in treatment of pocket where new tissues are formed and reattachment occurs as repair in areas of of root after surgical detachment.

122. CHEMICAL ANTIPLAQUE AGENTS

Mechanical plaque removal remains as the primary method used to prevent dental diseases and maintain oral health. However, chemical anti-plaque agents can be used to prevent (chemoprophylaxis) or treat (chemotherapy) the disease. These are divided into two groups:

1. Preventive agents that affect the development of supragingival plaque.
2. Therapeutic agents directed against subgingival plaque.

I. Oral Rinses

Advantages

a. High concentration of agent is delivered to local site.

b. Easy to use.

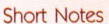
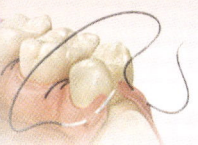

Disadvantages

a. Requires patient compliance.

b. Drug pulse and concentration limits the efficacy.

c. Limited to supragingival and mucosal areas.

Examples: Chlorhexidine (0.2%), essential oils.

II. Oral Irrigation

Advantages

a. Easy to use.

b. High concentration of agent delivered to local site.

c. Irrigates subgingival area.

Disadvantages

a. Requires patient dexterity and compliance.

b. Fluctuations in drug concentration are produced.

Examples: Plain water, chlorhexidine, essential oil and povidone iodine.

III. Local Drug Delivery System

Advantages

1. Reproduced and prolonged constant rate.

2. Less frequent administration.

3. Greater compliance

4. Fewer side effects.

5. Higher concentration achieved at local site.

6. Less patient variability.

Examples: Subgingivally delivered doxycycline, minocycline, chlorhexidine, etc.

Other chemical antiplaque agents include antibiotics, enzymes, quaternary ammonium compounds, etc.

123. CHLORHEXIDINE

The agent that has shown the most positive results, as anti-plaque agent is 0.2% chlorhexidine gluconate. Clinical studies have shown plaque reduction and more importantly gingivitis reduction. Chlorhexidine rinsing also reduces malodor.

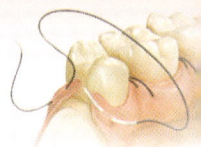

Mechanism of action of chlorhexidine:

1. The mechanism of action of chlorhexidine is based on the interaction of positive charged ions with negatively charged sites in the oral cavity.
2. Chlorhexidine molecule causes disruption of the bacterial cell membrane resulting in bacterial cell death, hence inhibits plaque formation.
3. Number of bacteria in the saliva available for adsorption to the teeth is significantly reduced.
4. Chlorhexidine molecules adsorb to the salivary glyco-proteins and prevent their adsorption to the tooth surface and the formation of acquired pellicle.
5. By coating the salivary bacteria with chlorhexidine mole-cules, adsorption of bacteria to the tooth surface is prevented.
6. By displacing calcium from the plaque components to-gether, chlorhexidine molecules disperse newly formed plaque thereby preventing plaque maturation and binding.
7. Chlorhexidine molecule causes disruption of the bacterial cell membrane resulting in bacterial cell death.

There are local, reversible side effects to chlorhexidine use primarily brown staining of teeth and transient impairment of taste perception.

124. DATUN AS AN ORAL HYGIENE AID

It is well established that plaque is the prime etiological factor in periodontal disease. In order to reduce the microbial colonization, this plaque should be removed daily either by mechanical or chemical means. Datun is one of the traditional mechanical plaque control aid.

Datun or the use of a twig is a practice for oral hygiene measure transmitted from father to son from time immemorial. The twig can either be of a Babool, Neem, or Banyan tree. It is reported that the fresh twig of "Nimva" was one of the best twigs used and the juice extracted by its chewing was believed to be beneficial for toning up the gums, and the chewing of any twig exercises the jaws. At the same time, it is observed that the use of datun produces unpleasant taste, mild gingivitis,

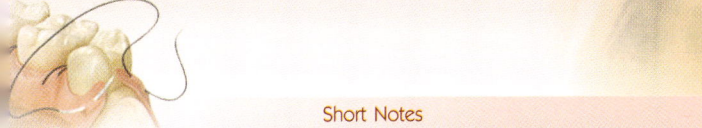

laceration of the gingiva and inability to reach all the areas of the mouth. This method is time consuming and did not make the mouth feel fresh. The fibers of the twig get between the teeth and it becomes difficult to remove. Comparing the effectiveness of datun and tooth brush as cleansing agent it is suggested that the tooth brush is superior to datun. Plaque removal by datun is significantly less than tooth brush and hence its use should be discouraged.

125. GINGIVAL MASSAGE

It is a procedure performed by the patient to make the gingiva firm and to increase cornification of the epithelium. It is one of the oral hygiene procedures and performed along with it. The objectives of gingival massage are: (1) To promote circulation, (2) To promote keratinization of the gingival epithelium, (3) To promote thickening of the epithelium, (4) To promote mitotic activity.

The massaging aids, which can be used by patients, are:
1. Interdental stimulator (plastic, rubber)
2. Rubber tip gingival stimulator
3. Balsa wood wedges (Stim-U-Dent)
4. Digital massage.

Massaging the gingiva, with a tooth brush, interdental cleansers or digital, produces epithelial thickening and increased mitotic activity. The increased keratinization and improved blood circulation may provide substantial protection against microorganisms and other local irritants and are, therefore, beneficial or necessary for gingival health.

126. TOOTHBRUSH—USES AND ABUSES

Toothbrush is the fundamental tool for the mechanical removal of plaque and other deposits.

The objectives of oral hygiene with tooth brush are as follows (uses):
1. To reduce the number of microorganisms on the teeth.
2. To promote circulation of the gingiva.
3. To promote cornification of the gingival (oral) epithelium

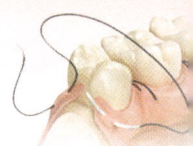

Abuses of toothbrush: Alterations in the gingiva as well as abrasions of the teeth may result from aggressive brushing in a horizontal or rotary fashion. The tooth brush trauma may be acute or chronic. The acute changes are varied in appearance and duration and include scuffing of the epithelium with denudation of the underlying connective tissue to form painful gingival bruise. Punctate lesions are produced by penetration of the gingiva by perpendicularly aligned bristles. Painful vesicle formation in traumatized areas is also seen. Diffuse erythema and denudation of the attached gingiva throughout the mouth may be a striking sequela of overzealous brushing. A toothbrush bristle forcibly embedded and retained in the gingiva is a common cause of the acute gingival abscess. Chronic toothbrush trauma results in gingival recession with denudation of the root surface. Often the gingival margin is enlarged and appears to be "piled up" as if it were molded in conformity with the strokes of the tooth brush. Linear grooves that extend from the marginal to the attached gingivae may be present.

127. SPECIFICATIONS OF A TOOTHBRUSH

The toothbrush is the fundamental tool for the mechanical removal of plaque and other deposits. Toothbrushes come in a variety of sizes, shapes, bristle-textures, length and bristle arrangement.

The American Dental Association has described the range of dimensions of acceptable brushes.

Toothbrushes should have a brushing surface from 1 to 1.25 inch (25.4 to 31.8 mm) long and 5/16 to 3/8 inch (7.9 to 9.5 mm) wide, two to four rows of bristles, and 5 to 12 tufts per row. Four row brushes contain more bristles and, therefore, tolerate more working pressure without flexing. Rounded bristle ends are assumed to be safer than flat cut bristles with sharp ends. Diameters of commonly used bristles range from 0.007 inch (0.2 mm) for soft brushes to 0.012 inch (0.3 mm) for medium brushes and 0.014 inch (0.4 mm) for hand brushes. Bass recommended a straight handle and nylon bristles 0.007 inch (0.2 mm) in diameter and inch 10.3 mm long with rounded

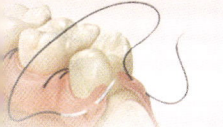

ends, arranged in three to four rows of tufts, six evenly spaced tufts per row with 80 to 86 bristles per tuft. For children, the brush is smaller with thinner (0.005 inch or 0.1 mm) and shorter 8.7 mm bristles.

128 FACTORS IN SELECTION OF A TOOTHBRUSH

The following points should be taken into consideration while selecting and recommending a toothbrush.

1. Proper brush should provide easy accessibility to all areas of the mouth. Small-headed brushes are often helpful in this regard.
2. Toothbrush should clean efficiently and be easy for the patient to manipulate.
3. In terms of homogeneity of the material, uniformity of bristle size, elasticity, resistance to fracture and repulsion of water and debris, nylon filaments are superior.
4. Multitufted brushes contain more bristles, so they clean more efficiently.
5. Rounded bristles cause less scratches on gingiva than flat cut bristles with sharp ends.

For the routine patients, a short-headed brush with straight cut round ended, soft to medium nylon bristles arranged in three or four rows of tufts is recommended. Toothbrush should be replaced after every 3 to 4 months.

129. BASS METHOD OF TOOTHBRUSHING

Bass method, if properly performed, is efficient at removing dental microbial plaque from the surfaces of the teeth, gingiva and from gingival sulcus. In this method, the bristles are directed into the gingival sulcus. A vibratory motion is then used to break-up the subgingival tooth-associated plaque as well as tissue-associated plaque colonies. Forty different tooth-brush positions are used to cover the full dentition.

On the facial and lingual surfaces of the posterior teeth, the head of the brush is placed parallel with the occlusal surfaces of the teeth and the bristles are directed apically into the gingival sulcus at a 45-degree angle to the long axes of the teeth.

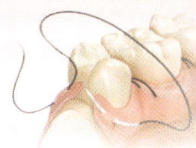

The toothbrush is activated by applying gentle pressure in an apical direction and by making short vibrating strokes, without lifting the toothbrush (Fig. 4.40). This forces the bristle ends into the gingival sulci and interproximal embrasures. It should produce perceptible blanching of the gingiva.

On the lingual surfaces of the anterior teeth, it is recommended that the brush be placed in a vertical direction parallel with the long axis of the teeth and only one or two teeth be brushed at a time.

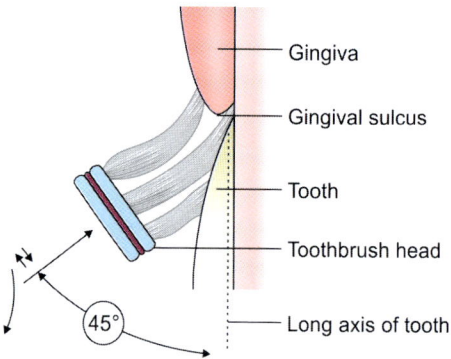

Fig. 4.40: Modified Bass technique

Occlusal surfaces: Press the bristles firmly on the occlusal surfaces with the ends as deeply as possible into the pits and fissures. Activate the brush with 20 short back, and, forth strokes until all posterior teeth are cleaned.

Modified Bass method: The modification consists of sweeping the bristles downward or upward over the tooth surface occlusally after completing the vibratory or back-and-forth motion in the gingival sulcus.

130. MODIFIED STILLMAN METHOD OF TOOTHBRUSHING

The soft or medium multitufted brush is used. The brush should be placed with the bristle ends resting partly on the cervical portion of the teeth and partly on the adjacent gingiva; pointing apically at an oblique angle to the long axis of the teeth

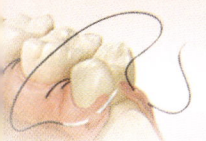

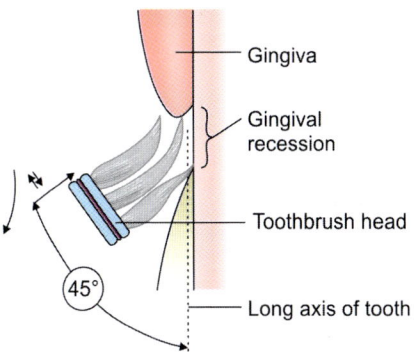

- Gingiva
- Gingival recession
- Toothbrush head
- 45°
- Long axis of tooth

Fig. 4.41: Modified Stillman method

(Fig. 4.41). The brush is activated 20 short back-and-forth strokes and moved in a coronal direction, along the attached gingiva, gingival margin and the tooth surface. This process is repeated on all the tooth surfaces.

This method of toothbrushing is recommended for cleaning the areas with gingival recession and root exposure.

131. CHARTERS TOOTHBRUSHING METHOD

The Charters method may be used when the interdental papillae do not fill the embrasure spaces or with open inter-proximal embrasure spaces. This technique provides a greater potential for gingival massage and after periodontal surgery.

A soft to medium, multi-tufted brush is placed on the teeth with the bristles pointed toward the crown at a 45-degree angle to the long axis of the teeth. The sides of the bristles are flexed against the gingiva and back-and-forth vibratory motion is used (Fig. 4.42). To cleanse the occlusal surfaces, the bristle tips are placed in the pits and fissures and the brush is activated with short back-and-forth strokes. The surfaces are cleansed segment by segment.

This method is especially suitable for gingival massage. When used with soft toothbrush, this technique can be recommended for temporary cleaning in areas for healing wounds following periodontal surgery.

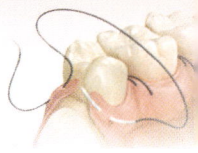

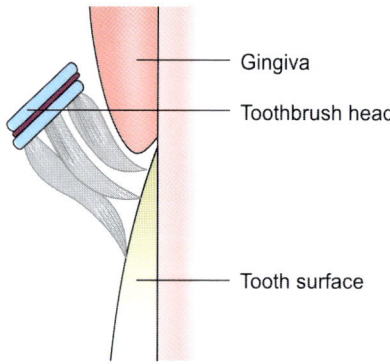

Gingiva

Toothbrush head

Tooth surface

Fig. 4.42: Charters method

132 FONES TOOTHBRUSHING METHOD

The brush is pressed firmly against the teeth and gingiva with the handle parallel to the line of occlusion and the bristles perpendicular to the facial tooth surfaces. The brush is then moved in a rotary motion with the teeth in occlusion up to the mucobuccal fold. This method is useful especially for young children and beginners.

133. POWERED TOOTHBRUSHES

Toothbrushes which use the electric power to move the head of the brush in either oscillating or rotatory motion are powered toothbrushes. Recently, ultrasonic toothbrushes are also developed.

Powered toothbrushes work primarily by contacting between the bristle and the tooth to remove the plaque. The oscillations or rotations loosen the bacterial plaque.

Number of studies comparing manual and powered toothbrushes failed to establish the benefits of powered toothbrush in longer duration. These have been shown to improve the oral health status in:

1. Children with mental and/or physical disabilities.
2. Hospitalized patients.
3. Patients with orthodontic appliances.

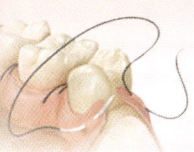

However, for well-motivated individuals or chronic periodontitis patients, it did not show any additional benefits.

134. INTERPROXIMAL (INTERDENTAL) CLEANING AIDS

The need for regular removal of plaque from the interproximal tooth surface is emphasized by the fact that the most frequent site of periodontal disease is in the interdental periodontal tissue. Toothbrushing is not usually effective for the removal of interproximal plaque and materia alba. Due to this, various aids have been developed for cleaning interproximal areas. The use and selection of these aids depend on the clinical characteristics of the embrasure spaces, the condition of the gingival tissues, and the patient's need.

Dental floss: For patients who have healthy periodontal tissues with no gingival recession, dental floss provides maximal access and cleaning effectiveness for flat or convex proximal tooth surfaces. Several types of dental floss are available.

Other Interdental Cleansing Devices

Wooden or rubber tips: The toothpick is made of a soft wood and is triangular in shape to contour the interdental spaces to remove microbial plaque. It is contraindicated for areas where the interdental papillae fill the interdental gingival embrasure spaces.

Rubber tips: These are placed in the interdental space in such a way that the base of the triangle rests on the gingiva and the sides are in contact with the proximal tooth surfaces. It is then repeatedly moved in and out of the embrasure, removing soft deposits from the teeth and mechanically stimulating the papillary gingiva.

Perio-aid: Wooden toothpick can be attached to a handle, such as perio-aid. It is used on facial and lingual surfaces throughout the mouth. Either sides or tip of the tooth pick is particularly efficient for cleaning along gingival margin and into periodontal pockets.

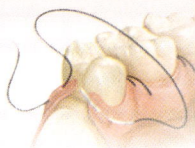

Interdental brushes: Small cone-shaped or tapered brushes are particularly helpful in cleaning large open interdental embrasure spaces and furcations. These brushes can adapt easily to irregular and concave tooth surfaces. They are inserted interproximally and are activated with short back-and-forth strokes in between the teeth. For best cleaning efficiency, the diameter of the toothbrush should be slightly larger than the gingival embrasures so that the bristles can exert pressure on the tooth surfaces working their way into the concavities of the root surfaces.

135. DENTAL FLOSS

Dental flossing is the most widely, recommended method of cleaning proximal tooth surfaces. Dental floss provides maximal access and cleaning effectiveness for flat or convex proximal tooth surfaces. Floss is available as multifilament nylon yarn that is twisted or non-twisted, bonded or non-bonded, waxed or un-waxed and thick or thin and monofilament or multifilament. Recommendations about type of floss should be based on ease of use and personal preference.

There are several ways of using dental floss. The floss must contact the proximal surface from line angle to line angle in order to clean effectively. A piece of floss long enough, i.e. 12–18 inches, should be grasped securely. It should be wrapped around the fingers or the ends may be tied together in a loop (Fig. 4.43). The floss should be stretched tightly between the thumb and the forefinger, or between both forefingers and

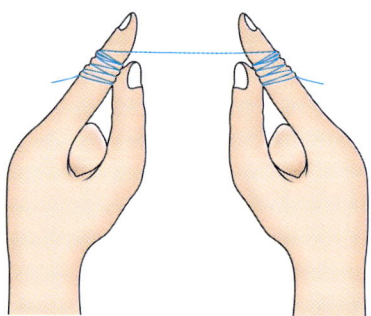

Fig. 4.43: Floss holding method

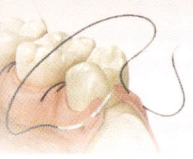

passed gently through each contact area with a firm back-and-forth motion. Wrap the floss around the proximal surface of one tooth, and slip it to the base of the gingival sulcus. Move the floss firmly along the tooth up to the contact area and gently down into the sulcus again, repeating this up and down stroke two or three times. Move the floss across the interdental gingiva and repeat the procedure on the proximal surface of the adjacent tooth. Continue the procedure throughout till the distal surface of the last tooth.

Flossing can be made easier by using a floss holder (Fig.4.44).

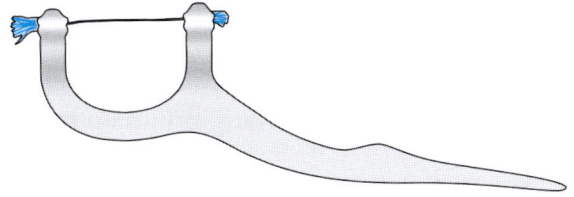

Fig. 4.44: Floss holder

Floss holders are useful:

a. For patients lacking manual dexterity.
b. For nursing personnel who assist handicapped and hospitalized patients.

The purpose of flossing is to remove plaque, not to dislodge fibrous threads of food wedged in between two teeth. Dental floss is recommended in type I embrasures.

136. THE GINGIVAL EMBRASURES

When adjacent teeth are in contact, the spaces that widen out from the contact are known as embrasures. Embrasures are of critical considerations in restorative dentistry. Proximal surfaces of dental restorations are important.as they create the embrasures for gingival health. There are 4 types—a facial, a lingual, an occlusal or incisal embrasure, and a gingival. In the healthy state, the gingival embrasure is filled with soft tissue, but in periodontal disease, spaces are created in the gingival embrasure.

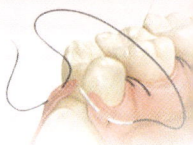

Periodontal disease causes tissue destruction, which reduces the level of the alveolar bone, increases the size of the gingival embrasure, and creates open interdental space.

Dimensions of Gingival Embrasures

Height: The distance between the contact area and the bone margin.

Width: The distance mesiodistally between the proximal surfaces.

Depth: The distance faciolingually from the contact area to a line joining the proximofacial/proximolingual line angles.

Three types of interproximal embrasures can be distinguished (Fig. 4.45):

1. Type I embrasures—are totally occupied by the interdental papillae.
2. Type II embrasures—are characterized by slight to moderate recession of the interdental papillae.
3. Type III embrasures—are created by extensive recession or complete loss of interdental papillae.

The selection of the interdental cleansing aids should be according to the type of embrasure that exists in the patient's mouth.

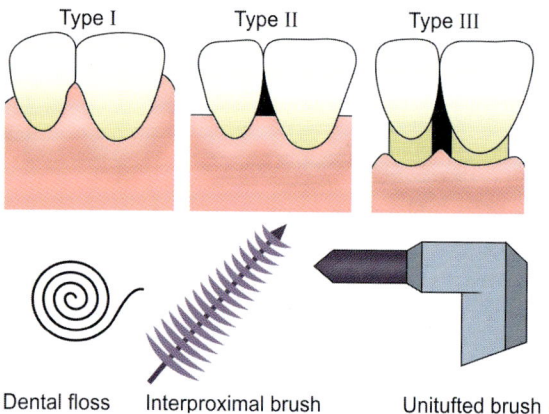

Fig. 4.45: Types of embrasures

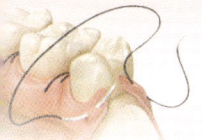

- In type I, dental floss is used—no gingival recession.
- In type II, interdental brush—moderate papillary recession.
- In type III, unitufted brush is used—complete loss of papillae.

137. DISCLOSING AGENTS

A patient generally knows that it is desirable to remove food debris, which are relatively easily seen or felt, but the need to remove, the more tenaciously attached colorless plaque, is not always recognized. Plaque is generally invisible and must be stained for patient's observation (Figs 4.46A and B). The purpose of the staining is to enable the patient to visualize the stained deposits so as to increase the effectiveness of plaque removal. In addition, the disclosing of plaque helps the patients

A

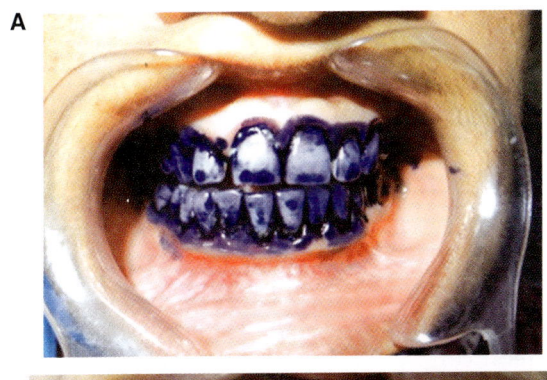

B

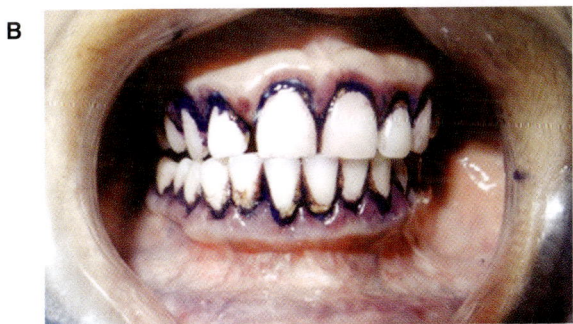

Fig. 4.46: (A) Disclosing agent application; (B) Disclosing agent after spitting

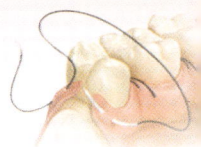

learn difference between bacterial dental plaque and food debris. Disclosing agents aid in patient education, motivation and home care because the patient can use these dyes or solutions to judge the effectiveness of the oral hygiene routine. The patient uses the disclosing agents at home to monitor personal progress. First the daily use is recommended and then periodically after the plaque removal techniques have been perfected.

These disclosing stains come in tablet, liquid and wafer forms. Wafers are crushed between the teeth and swished around the mouth for a few seconds and then spit out. Solutions are applied on to the teeth in concentrates on cotton swabs or as dilutes in mouthwashes. They usually produce heavy staining of bacterial plaque. They are water-soluble and stain plaque blue, purple or red depending on the type of stain used. Examples of disclosing solutions are Bismark brown solution, Basic fuschin solution, erythrosine (FDC red number) and sodium fluorescein dye.

138. IMPORTANCE OF PATIENT'S EDUCATION AND MOTIVATION IN PREVENTIVE PERIODONTICS

Education and motivation of the patient to take care of his own oral cavity are essential for effective prevention and control of periodontal disease. Daily personal care by the patient is perhaps more important. The finest work performed by the dental surgeon can be wasted, if the patient neglects to take care of his own mouth. The patient must be told and shown that periodontal disease is insidious and usually asymptomatic. Patients should be shown areas of gingivitis and stained plaque in their own mouths after disclosing solutions have been applied. They should be shown how to maneuver a toothbrush to clean all areas of the mouth, especially those areas that they have been missing. Patient's motivation requires frequent reinforcement. Therefore, every recall visit should include an evaluation of oral hygiene status and a comparison with the previous records. The oral hygiene habits should be encouraged and developed in the child as early as possible. To motivate patients to perform prescribed oral hygiene practices

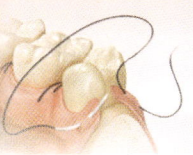

conscientiously and over a long period, requires time, patience and ingenuity. But unless the effort is successfully made, the treatment provided will, in large part, be rendered ineffective. To be successful in transferring the information to his patients in a convincing way, the dentist must be a firm believer in the importance of proper oral hygiene and must practice it conscientiously himself.

139. ORAL PHYSIOTHERAPY (ORAL HYGIENE)

The objective of oral hygiene is to reduce the number of microorganisms on the teeth. All accessible dental plaque and debris should be removed from gingival margins, proximal tooth surfaces, and where possible from gingival sulci. Doing this reduces the factors that produce irritation and inflammation. One of the causes of halitosis is also removed by these measures. Gingival stimulation (massage) may play a role in increasing gingival tone, surface keratinization, gingival vascularity, and gingival circulation.

Introducing an oral hygiene program to the patient is of high importance in every periodontal treatment plan. Plaque control instructions should begin at the first therapeutic appointment. The patient is taught how to clean all smooth and regular surfaces of the teeth.

The toothbrush is often the only hygiene aid indicated at this stage of therapy. Dental floss should be used on smooth proximal tooth surfaces only, because flossing around sharp edges and coarse surfaces of calculus or overhanging restorations causes the floss to shred and break. It leads to ineffective plaque removal, as well as persistence of inflammatory bleeding. It must be impressed upon dentulous individuals that it is their obligation to remove deposits consistently to prevent adverse tissue response. The primary cause of plaque accumulation is the lack of knowledge, skill, and desire on the part of the patient to remove such deposits. It is dental surgeon's duty to alter these three variables by proper oral physiotherapy, i.e. the procedures practiced by the patient for the purpose of maintaining good oral hygiene.

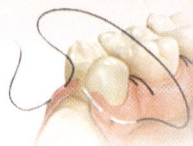

140. DOXYCYCLINE

Doxycycline is an antibiotic of group tetracycline derived semi-synthetically from certain species of *Streptomyces*. It is effective against broad-spectrum of microorganisms.

Advantages of doxycycline over tetracycline:

1. Patient compliance due to once daily dose.
2. Its absorption from the GI tract is slightly altered by calcium, metal ions or antacids.

Doxycycline in periodontics:

1. Doxycycline appears in gingival crevicular fluid soon after consumption. This allows a high drug concentration to be delivered into periodontal pocket.
2. Systemic doxycycline is effective against *A. actinomy-cetemcomitans* from tissue when used in conjunction with scaling and root planing.
3. The anti-collagenase activity of doxycycline can be used with sub-antimicrobial dose as host modulation therapy.
4. Doxycycline used as locally delivered drug in gel form was shown to be effective clinically.
    1. **Systemic:** 100 mg bid for the first day followed by 100 mg once daily for 21 days, e.g. Cap. Doxy IL.
    2. **Sub-antimicrobial:** 20 mg twice daily for longer duration depending upon the periodontal condition, e.g. Tab. Periostat.
    3. **Subgingival:** 10% doxycycline in gel form, e.g. Atridox.

141. METRONIDAZOLE IN PERIODONTAL THERAPY

Metronidazole is a nitroimidazole which is bactericidal to anaerobic organisms. It disrupts bacterial DNA synthesis in conditions of low reduction potential.

Indications: To treat:

a. Gingivitis
b. ANUG
c. Chronic periodontitis
d. Aggressive periodontitis
e. Refractory periodontitis when used in combination with amoxicillin.

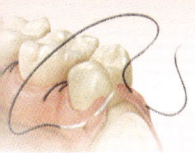

Metronidazole, like many other drugs, is effective only when used in combination with scaling and root planing and not as a monotherapy.

This drug is active against anaerobic organisms as antimicrobial agent. In conjunction with the pocket treatment, antimicrobial agents may be of importance in following ways:

1. Antimicrobials may be valuable in reaching and killing bacteria that cannot be removed by scaling, root planing, and curettage, e.g. bacteria that have penetrated into the tissues in advanced periodontitis, localized aggressive periodontitis, furcations, etc.

2. The use of antimicrobials in conjunction with non-surgical therapy may reduce or eliminate the indications for periodontal surgery. It may also be useful in increasing the interval between two recall maintenance visits.

One single dose of this drug (250 mg, oral) appears in both serum and gingival fluid in sufficient quantities to inhibit a wide range of suspected periodontal pathogens. Administered systemically (750 to 1000 mg per day for 2 weeks), this drug suppresses the growth of anaerobic flora, including spirochetes, and decreases the clinical and histopathologic signs of periodontitis.

142. CONSERVATIVE METHODS OF POCKET ELIMINATION

Scientific criteria to establish the indications for each or different techniques or methods are difficult to determine. Clinical experience, however, has suggested the criteria for selecting the method to be used to eliminate the pocket in individual cases. The conservative methods for pocket elimination depend on various factors, such as (i) type of pocket, (ii) consistency of the gingiva, (iii) age of the patient, (iv) depth of the pocket and (v) etiological factor.

Microbial plaque and other local irritants cause gingival inflammation and pocket formation. The pockets which are formed may be of gingival type or periodontal type. In association with pocket formation, at times the consistency of the gingiva also changes from fibrotic to edematous.

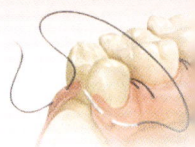

The supragingival, subgingival scaling and root planing help in removing the local irritants, thereby reducing or totally eliminating the pocket depth. This is possible when the pocket wall is edematous and there is accessibility.

Application of certain caustic agents on the inner side (lateral wall of the pocket) of the pocket wall of the gingiva would cause shrinkage of edematous tissue and hence elimination of the pocket. Placement of local drug delivery agent to infection sites is also effective for reduction of pocket.

Gingival curettage helps in removing the pathology within the pocket wall of the gingiva which results in elimination of the pocket.

Proper oral hygiene methods with proper aids help in reducing the pathological deepened sulcus.

143. ROOT PLANING

It is the procedure by which residual embedded calculus and diseased cementum are removed from the roots to produce a smooth, clean, hard surface.

The purpose of root planing is to eliminate the etiologic agents, subgingival plaque and its products from the tooth surface to restore gingival health. It contains concealed spicules of calculus covered by plaque, which initiates the inflammatory process and promotes deepening of the pocket.

Root surfaces exposed to plaque and calculus, pose a different problem. Deposits of calculus on root surfaces are frequently embedded in cemental irregularities, scaling alone is, therefore, insufficient to remove them. A portion of the cementum itself must be removed to eliminate these deposits. Furthermore, when cementum is exposed to plaque and the pocket environment, its surface is contaminated by toxic substances, notably endotoxins. This altered cementum is a source of gingival irritation and must be removed by root planing to produce a hard, clean surface that is free of toxic substances.

Subgingival scaling and root planing should not be thought of or practiced as separate procedures. It is apparent that scaling without root planing will often be inadequate to remove all the factors responsible for gingival inflammation, from root surfaces.

144. LOCAL DRUG DELIVERY AGENTS

Locally delivered antimicrobial agents are adjuncts to scaling and root planing to control the growth of bacteria. These are as follows:

1. **Tetracycline containing fibers:** Tetracycline fiber of 0.5 mm diameter packed into periodontal pocket was well tolerated and reduced probing depth, bleeding on probing and provided gain in clinical attachment level (Fig. 4.47B).

2. **Subgingival doxycycline:** A gel system in a syringe with 10% doxycycline (Atridox) is available. It was the only local delivery system accepted by the American Dental Association (ADA). Treatment with 10% doxycycline gel alone was found to be more effective than the other treatments.

3. **Subgingival minocycline:** A locally delivered sustained release minocylcline (Arestin) is available for subgingival placement as an adjunct to scaling and root planing. 2% minocycline is encapsulated into bioresorbable microspheres in a gel carrier. There was improvement in all the clinical parameters and increase in clinical attachment levels in patients with 5 to 7 mm pocket depths.

4. **Subgingival chlorhexidine:** A resorbable delivery system of chlorhexidine gluconate (periochip) has shown positive clinical results (Fig. 4.47A). Periochip is small chip composed of a biodegradable hydrolysed gelatin matrix, cross-linked with glutaraldehyde, glycerine and water, into which 2.5 mg of chlorhexidine gluconate has been incorporated. The delivery system releases chlorhexidine for at least 7 days, concentrations well above the tolerance of most bacteria. The chip biodegrades in 7 to 10 days hence removal is not required.

5. **Subgingival metronidazole:** Topical medication containing an oil-based metronidazole (25%) gel has been tested. Subgingival metronidazole demonstrated equivalent efficacy as that of scaling and root planing.

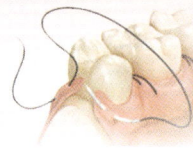

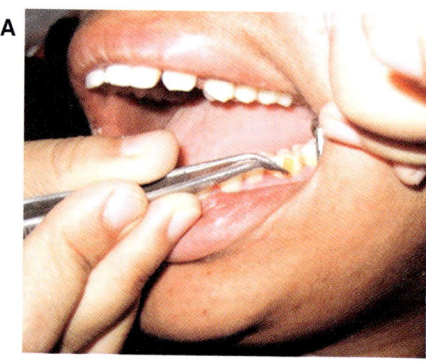

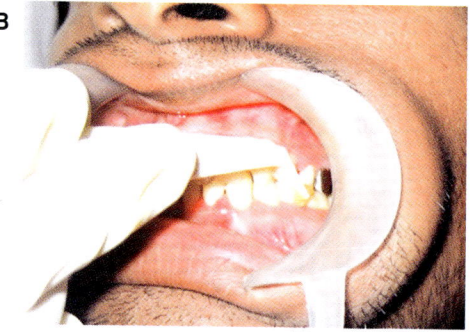

Fig. 4.47: (A) Chlorhexidine chip; (B) Tetracycline fibers

145. HOST MODULATION THERAPY (HMT)

These are the therapeutic modalities used to alter the function or status of the host so as to improve the outcome of the therapy, slow down the progression of the disease and allow for more predictable management of patients.

HMT is used as an adjunct to conventional therapy especially in refractory cases. HMT focuses on alteration in the inflammatory response, such as:

I. Inhibition of matrix metalloproteinase, and
II. Limit the inflammatory effect of prostanoids and cytokines.

This can be achieved by systemically or locally delivered drugs. A variety of agents have been evaluated as host modulating agents:

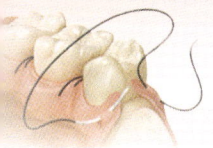
1. **NSAIDs:** Inhibition of prostaglandin E2 systemic as well as local administration.

   Systemic: Salicylate, propionic acid derivatives (e.g. ibuprofen)

   Local: Ketorolac mouthwash.

2. **Bisphosphonates:** Bone seeking agents inhibit bone resorption and possess anti-collagenase properties.

3. **Subantimicrobial-dose-doxycycline (SDD):** Low dose doxycycline (20 mg twice daily for 3 months) is indicated as HMT. It exerts its effect by inhibition of enzymes, cytokines and osteoclasts.

4. **Local administration of enamel matrix proteins, growth factors, bone morphogenetic proteins:** These agents are helpful in improving healing and stimulation of regeneration of lost periodontal structures.

146. INTERDISCIPLINARY PERIODONTICS (MULTIDISCIPLINARY PERIODONTICS)

Cooperation, coordination and interaction between different specialties in dentistry are extremely important in establishing diagnosis and treatment planning for a successful therapy. An appropriate identification of causes, proper sequencing and performance of treatment is critical. Therefore, the role of various disciplines and their relationship with periodontics should not be overlooked.

A. Restorative Dentistry and Periodontics

1. Material used for restorations should not be harmful for periodontal tissues.

2. Biologic width should not be violated while placing the margins of the restorations.

3. Contours of restorations should be such that it maintains the self-cleansing areas.

4. Occlusal harmony should be established.

5. Ideal embrasures should be created so as to avoid food impaction and to enhance esthetics.

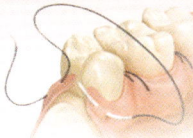

B. Endodontics and Periodontics

Endo-Perio lesions are of following types:

1. Primary endodontic lesion only.
2. Primary endodontic lesion with secondary periodontal involvement.
3. Primary periodontal lesion only.
4. Primary periodontal lesion with secondary endodontic involvement.
5. True combined lesions.

Pulp and periodontal communication can occur through apical foramina, accessory canals, dentinal tubules, developmental grooves or root anomalies.

Clinical Considerations

1. Pulp necrosis can result in resorption of periapical bone and treatment of infected pulp (RCT) can recover it.
2. Periodontitis rarely produces pulpal changes, but when the involvement of pulp occurs with primary periodontal lesion, treatment of endodontic lesion first followed by periodontal treatment would give excellent results.

C. Orthodontics and Periodontics

Often periodontal health is improved by orthodontic treatment and orthodontic tooth movement is often facilitated by periodontal therapy.

Clinical Considerations

1. Malaligned teeth, such as crowding, deep bite, etc., favor plaque accumulation which in turn can lead to periodontal disease. Minor orthodontic corrections can be carried out in phase I periodontal therapy, would help to improve the resultant outcome.
2. Patient undergoing orthodontic treatment should be under supervision of a periodontist so as to diagnose and eliminate the initial periodontal disease.
3. Periodontally accelerated osteogenic orthodontics (PAOO/ rapid orthodontics/wilckodontics): To accelerate the tooth

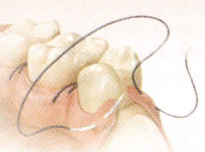

movement in orthodontics, a periodontal surgery with osteoplasty is performed, to prepare the alveolar bone for desired tooth movement. This facilitates the tooth movements thereby reducing the period of orthodontic treatment nearly by half.

147. BIOLOGIC WIDTH

Biologic width is the space occupied by healthy gingival tissue coronal to the crest of the alveolar bone which includes junctional epithelium (approx. 1 mm) and connective tissue attachment (approx 1 mm). It is relatively constant (2 mm$^{+/-}$ 30%) (Fig. 4.48).

Clinical implication: Biologic width should not be violated while placing the restoration margins. Margins of the restoration should be placed into the gingival sulcus and at least 2 mm away from the alveolar bone. If not, the gingival tissue will be inflamed with no other evident etiological factor.

Violation of biologic width interproximally, can be identified on radiographs and can be corrected by:

1. Surgically removing the bone away from proximity to the margins of restorations.

2. Orthodontically extruding the tooth.

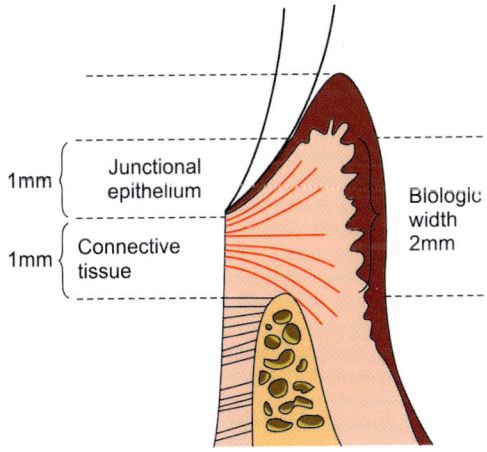

Fig. 4.48: Biologic width

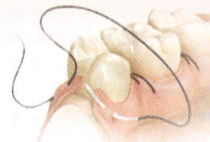

148 GENERAL PRINCIPLES OF PERIODONTAL SURGERY

1. **Patients preparation:**

   Re-evaluation after phase I therapy

   Premedication: Pre-surgical medications of antibiotics and NSAIDs can be advocated.

   Smoking: Patient should discontinue smoking 3–4 weeks after procedure.

   Informed consent: It should be obtained verbally as well as in writing prior to surgery.

2. **Emergency equipment:** All auxiliaries and operator should be trained to handle all possible emergencies that may arise during procedure. Emergency drugs and equipment should be readily available.

3. **Prevention of transmission of infection:** Universal aseptic and sterilization precautions should be followed to prevent the disease transmission.

4. **Sedation and anesthesia:** Periodontal surgery should be performed painlessly which requires effective administration of local anesthesia along with sedative agents, if required.

5. **Tissue management:** Surgery should be performed without having trauma to the tissue. For this, tissue should be handled carefully and instruments should be sharp.

6. **Scaling and root planing:** Rough areas/calculus should be checked and removed, if present.

7. **Hemostasis:** Routinely, hemostasis will occur after removal of granulation tissue. If tissues are handled carefully and gently, less bleeding will occur. If a bleeder is located, adrenaline pressure pack is given, laser beam is applied or the vessel can be ligated.

   For slow, constant blood flow or oozing, hemostasis may be achieved by applying hemostatic agent, such as absorbable gelatin sponge or oxidized cellulose.

8. **Periodontal dressing:** It can be applied to protect the tissue thereby assisting healing.

9. **Postoperative instructions:** Should be given verbally as well as in writing.

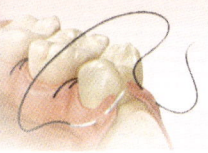

149. HOSPITAL PERIODONTAL SURGERY

Periodontal surgery is routinely performed as clinical procedure, sextant or quadrantwise at weekly, bi-weekly or longer intervals. But sometimes, according to patient's need full mouth surgery can be performed in single seating in operation theatre under general anesthesia. This is referred as *hospital periodontal surgery*. When general anesthesia is used, periodontal dressing should be placed after the sufficient recovery of the patient demonstrated by coughing reflex.

Indications

1. Apprehensive patient
2. Patients who cannot come for multiple visits to complete surgical treatment.
3. Patients with certain systemic conditions in whom special precautions are required, which can be best provided in hospital settings. The purpose of hospitalization is to protect the patients by anticipating their special needs.

150. INDICATIONS AND CONTRAINDICATIONS FOR SUBGINGIVAL CURETTAGE

Subgingival curettage: It refers to the procedure that is performed apical to the junctional epithelium, in which the connective tissue attachment is severed down to the osseous crest (Fig. 4.49).

Aim of curettage: To reduce pocket depth by:

a. Enhancing gingival shrinkage.
b. Enhancing new connective tissue attachment.

Indications

1. Subgingival curettage is indicated when a gingival inflammation persists after careful and thorough root planing with suprabony pockets and edematous gingival consistency.
2. Indicated in deep isolated infrabony pockets as part of new attachment attempts in moderately deep infrabony pockets inaccessible areas.

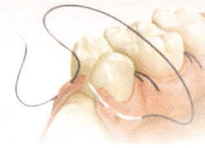

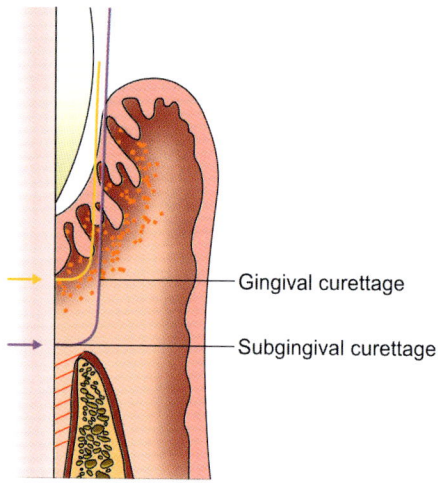

— Gingival curettage

— Subgingival curettage

Fig. 4.49: Curettage

3. Indicated in treatment of pockets when esthetics is given importance.

4. Indicated in patients, where other surgical procedures cannot be performed, due to advanced age, systemic and psychological problems.

5. Curettage is frequently performed on recall visits as a method of maintenance treatment for areas with recurrent inflammation and pocket depth, where pocket reduction surgery has previously been performed.

6. Shallow, infrabony pockets.

Contraindications

Subgingival curettage is contraindicated in cases:

1. Where the pocket wall of the gingiva is fibrotic.

2. Where the pockets are tortuous and intraalveolar.

3. Where the pockets are approaching mucogingival junction or apical to mucogingival junction.

4. Where the surgery of any type is contraindicated due to systemic problems.

151. EXCISIONAL NEW ATTACHMENT PROCEDURE (ENAP)

Indications

1. Suprabony pockets
2. Adequate keratinized tissue
3. When esthetic is an unimportant factor.

Contraindications

1. Pockets exceed mucogingival junction
2. Edematous tissue
3. Lack of keratinized tissue
4. Osseous defects have to be treated or are present.

Technique (Fig. 4.50)

1. After anesthesia, an internal bevel incision is made with a surgical blade from the margin of free gingiva apically to the point below the bottom of the pocket.
2. Inner portion of the soft tissue wall of the pocket is cut all around the tooth.
3. Excised tissue is removed with a curette. Root planing is done preserving all the connective tissue fibers attached to the root surface.

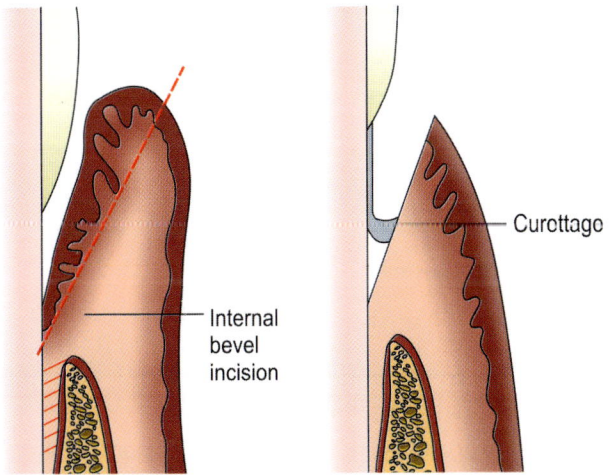

Internal bevel incision

Curettage

Fig. 4.50: ENAP

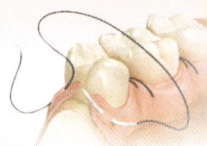

4. After good adaptation of the wound edges, sutures are placed and periodontal dressing is given.

The excisional new attachment procedure is an attempt to overcome some of the limitations of closed gingival curettage and gain new attachment in areas of true periodontal pockets. The ENAP, unlike scaling and curettage is a technique to ensure complete removal of sulcular epithelium, epithelial attachment, granulated and soft inflamed connective tissue, subgingival calculus, and softened cementum.

It is curettage with a surgical blade.

152. GINGIVECTOMY

Gingivectomy means excision of the diseased pocket wall along with complete removal of surface deposits and thorough root planing.

Indications

1. Elimination of suprabony pockets
2. Fibrous and firm pocket wall
3. Suprabony periodontal abscess.

Procedure (Fig. 4.51)

Step 1: Marking the pockets: After adequate anesthesia, pockets are measured and marked at its deepest point with a pocket marker at several areas of each surface; so as to get the bleeding points.

Step 2: Gingivectomy incisions: Incisions are taken with Kirkland gingivectomy knives or Bard Parker blades along with orban periodontal knives.

The incision is taken apical to the bleeding points joining all the bleeding points and is directed coronally. It should be as close as possible to the bone without exposing it, remove the pocket wall coronal to the bone.

The incision should be beveled at approximately 45 degrees angle to tooth surface, so as to create normal festooned pattern of the gingiva.

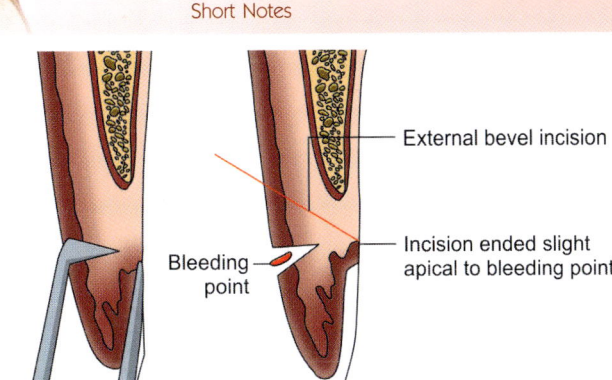

External bevel incision

Incision ended slight apical to bleeding point

Bleeding point

Pocket marker

Fig. 4.51: Gingivectomy

Step 3: Degranulation and root planing: Remove the excised pocket wall, clean and examine the area of the root surface.

Step 4: Curettage: Carefully curette the granulation tissue and remove remaining calculus and necrotic cementum.

Step 5: Dressing: Cover the area with a periodontal dressing.

The gingivectomy may be performed by means of scalpels, electrodes, lasers or chemicals.

153. GINGIVOPLASTY

It is the surgical reshaping of the gingiva to create physiologic gingival contours. Its sole purpose is recontouring the gingiva in the absence of pockets. Gingivoplasty can be performed without gingivectomy as a procedure in its own right when the gingival margins are blunt and fibrotic and when the pocket depth is minimal, pseudo pockets are present or in the absence of pockets (Fig. 4.52).

Gingival and periodontal disease often produces deformities in the gingiva that interfere with normal food excursion, collect irritating plaque and food debris, which prolong and aggravate the disease process. Gingival clefts, craters and shelf-like interdental papillae caused by acute necrotizing ulcerative

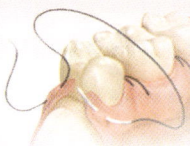

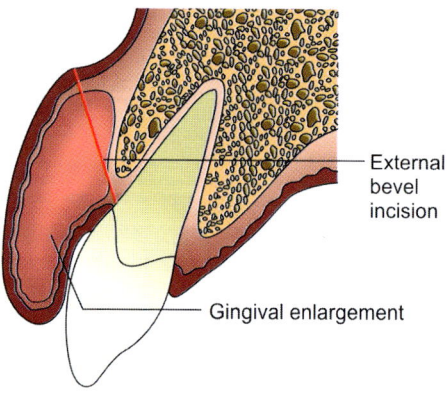

External
bevel
incision

Gingival enlargement

Fig. 4.52: Gingivoplasty

gingivitis and gingival enlargement are examples of such deformities.

The gingivoplasty technique is similar to the gingivectomy technique, its purpose, however, is different.

Gingivoplasty may be done with a periodontal knife, a Bard-Parker handle with blade, rotary coarse diamond stones, or electrodes.

It consists of procedures that resemble those performed in festooning artificial dentures, namely, tapering the gingival margin, creating an escalloped marginal outline, thinning the attached gingiva, and creating vertical interdental grooves and shaping the interdental papillae to provide sluice ways for the passage of food.

154. HEALING AFTER GINGIVECTOMY

Healing after Surgical Gingivectomy

1. There is formation of a protective surface blood clot and the underlying tissue becomes acutely inflamed.
2. The clot is replaced by granulation tissue and by 24 hours there is an increase in new connective tissue cells.
3. After 12 to 24 hours, epithelial cells at the margins of the wound start to migrate over the granulation tissue separating it from the contaminated surface layer of the clot.

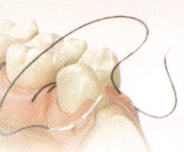

4. By the third day, number of fibroblasts are located in the area. The highly vascular granulation tissue grows coronally, creating a new free gingival margin and sulcus. Capillaries derived from blood vessels of the periodontal ligament migrate into the granulation tissue.

5. Surface epithelialization is generally complete after 5 to 14 days. During the first 4 weeks after gingivectomy, keratinization is less than it was prior to surgery.

6. Complete epithelial repair takes about one month.

7. Complete repair of the connective tissue takes about 7 weeks. The process of healing after gingivectomy is by secondary intention.

155. MERITS AND DEMERITS OF ELECTROSURGERY

Electrosurgery refers to the use of high frequency electric currents for cutting and destroying tissue. Some operators prefer to use electrosurgery for gingivectomy/gingivoplasty. This method employs either bipolar electrocoagulation or single wire electrodes. Both can be used as adjuncts to the knife, especially in areas where access is limited and difficult.

Merits

i. Electrosurgery is useful in cases where gingivoplasty is difficult to perform in an isolated area.

ii. Electrosurgery permits an adequate contouring of the tissue.

iii. It controls hemorrhage.

iv. It is time saving.

Demerits

i. Electrosurgery cannot be used in patients who have a non-compatible or a poorly shielded cardiac pacemaker.

ii. Treatment causes an unpleasant odor.

iii. Heat generated by electrosurgery may cause tissue damage and loss of periodontal support and bone.

iv. The healing after electrosurgery is delayed.

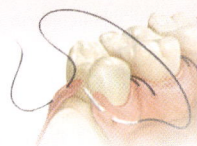

v. In gingivectomy procedure, it is difficult with electro-surgery to maintain proper bevel.

vi. Gingival recession.

vii. Bone necrosis, sequestration and loss of bone height (when used close to the bone)

viii. Furcations exposure.

156. FRENECTOMY

A frenum becomes a problem, if its attachment is too close to the marginal gingiva. It may then pull on healthy gingiva and invite the accumulation of irritants. It may deflect the wall of a periodontal pocket and aggravate its severity, or it may interfere with post-treatment healing. Frenal problems occur most often on the facial surface between maxillary and mandibular central incisors and in the canine and premolar areas.

Frenectomy is complete removal of the frenum, including its attachment to underlying bone. It may be required in the correction of an abnormal diastema between maxillary central incisors.

Frenectomy procedure depends upon the requirement, if the vestibule is deep enough, the operation is confined to the frenum only, but it is often necessary to deepen the vestibule to provide space for the repositioned frenum.

High frenal attachments on the lingual surface are uncommon.

Procedure for Frenectomy (Figs 4.53A to D)

1. Anesthetize the area.
2. Frenum is engaged with a hemostat inserted to the depth of the vestibule.
3. Incision is made along the upper surface of the hemostat, extending beyond the tip.
4. A similar incision is made along the undersurface of the hemostat.
5. A triangular portion of the frenum is removed.
6. A horizontal incision is made separating the fibers.

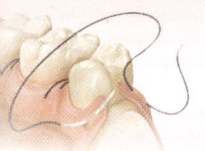

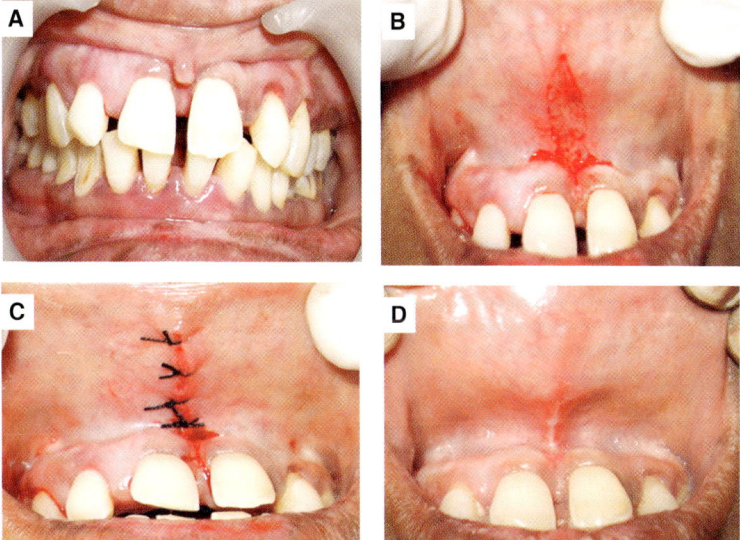

Fig. 4.53: Frenectomy:(A) Preoperative: high frenum; (B) Removal of frenum; (C) Suturing; (D) Postoperative: relocated frenum

7. Then labial mucosa is sutured to the apical periosteum.
8. Cleaning of the field of operation is done and packing with gauze sponges is done till bleeding stops.
9. Area is covered with dry foil and dressing is applied.

157. CROWN LENGTHENING PROCEDURES

 When a tooth has a short clinical crown that is inadequate for the retention of a required cast restoration, it is necessary to increase the size of the clinical crown using periodontal surgical procedures. These crown lengthening procedures provide an adequate area for crown retention without extending the crown margins deep into the periodontal tissues.

Clinical crown is that portion of the tooth that is coronal to the alveolar crest. Therefore, to lengthen it either marginal gingiva or the bone margin has to be removed. This is done with gingivectomy or apically displaced flap and ostectomy, which means that tooth supporting bone is removed. It is

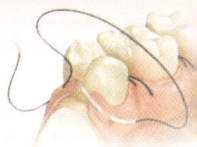

essential that there be at least 3 mm between the most apical extension of the restoration margin and the alveolar bone crest thereby maintaining the biologic width. This space allows sufficient room for the supracrestal collagen fibers that are part of the periodontal support mechanisms, as well as providing a gingival sulcus of 2 to 3 mm. Failure to allow sufficient space between the crown margin and the alveolar crest height means that the finished restoration is positioned deep in the periodontal tissues leading to inflammation and pocket formation.

158. CLASSIFICATION AND INDICATIONS OF PERIODONTAL FLAP

Periodontal flap is a section of gingiva and or mucosa surgically separated from the underlying tissues to provide visibility of and access to the bone and root surface.

Classification of Flaps

I. **Based on bone exposure after reflection:**

  a. *Full thickness*: All the soft tissue and periosteum are reflected to expose bone (Fig. 4.54).

  b. *Split thickness*: Only the epithelium and a layer of connective tissue are reflected (Fig. 4.55).

II. **Based on flap placement after surgery:**

  a. *Repositioned*: Positioned, or displaced flaps

  b. *Unrepositioned*: Non-displaced flaps.

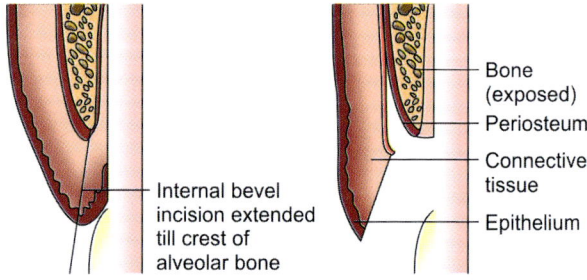

Fig. 4.54: Full thikness flap

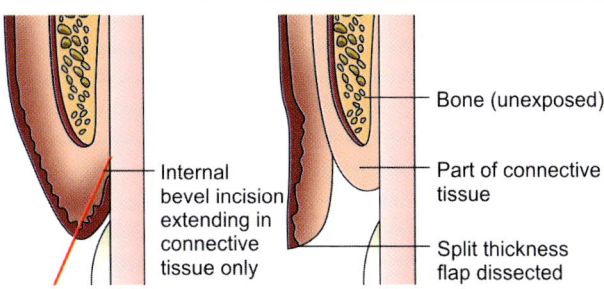

Bone (unexposed)

Internal
bevel incision
extending in
connective
tissue only

Part of connective
tissue

Split thickness
flap dissected

Fig. 4.55: Partial thickness flap

III. Based on the management of papilla:
   a. *Conventional*
   b. *Papilla preservation*

IV. Based on vertical incision:
   a. *Flap with vertical releasing incision*
   b. *Envelope flap*

Indications

Flap is indicated:

1. Where and when access to and visualization of the subgingival portion of the roots and bone is essential or required as a treatment procedure.
2. When flap requires manipulation for its desired positional goals.
3. When the periodontal pockets are of infrabony type with osseous defects.
4. In conditions when the periodontal pockets are close or apical to mucogingival junction.
5. In cases of isolated gingival recession of narrow type. In such cases, the flap which is indicated is partial thickness, displaced type of flap.

   Flap procedures seek to gain esthetic and structural goals in addition to pocket elimination.

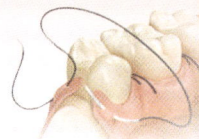

159. INCISIONS USED IN PERIODONTICS

For periodontal flaps horizontal and vertical incisions are used.

Horizontal Incisions

A. Internal bevel incision (first/reverse bevel incision): No. 15 surgical blade is used to make the incision. The incision is made 0.5 to 1 mm away from the gingival margin to the alveolar crest (Fig. 4.56).

Advantages

1. Pocket lining is removed along with the incision.
2. Relatively healthy gingival tissue is preserved.
3. Better adaptation of flap over bone produces sharp and thin margins.

B. Crevicular incision (second incision): It is made from the base of the pocket to the crest of the bone (Fig. 4.56).

First and second incisions together form a V-shaped wedge of the tissue attached to the crest of the bone.

C. Interdental incision (third incision): For this incision, Orban's knife is usually used. The incision is made facially, lingually as well as interdentally, to free the gingiva completely around tooth (Fig. 4.56).

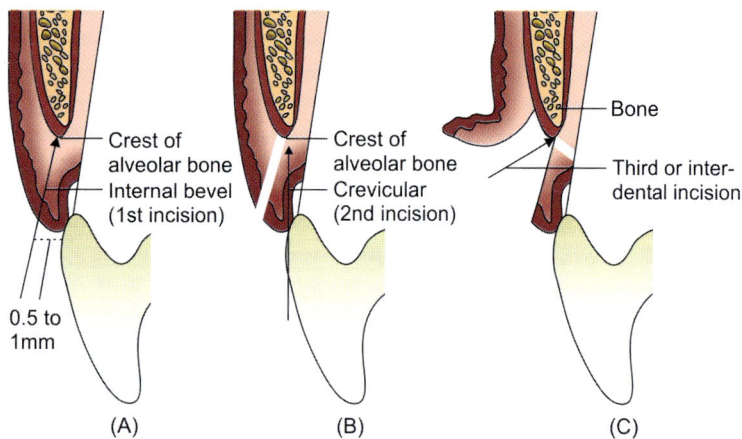

Fig. 4.56: Horizontal incisions

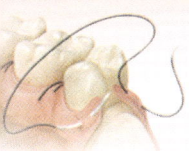
These three incisions together remove the pocket lining along with adjacent granulomatous tissue.

D. **Vertical incisions:** It can be placed on one or both the ends of horizontal incision which should extend beyond the mucogingival junction to release the flap adequately so that it can be displaced.

Vertical incision should be given at the line angels of the tooth either to include or exclude the papilla completely (Fig. 4.57). It should not be taken at the crest of the papilla. Vertical incision, if taken on both the ends of horizontal incision, should be placed obliquely to have broad base to maintain the blood supply of the flap.

Vertical incisions on palatal or lingual sides are avoided. Flap reflected without vertical incision is called "Envelope Flap".

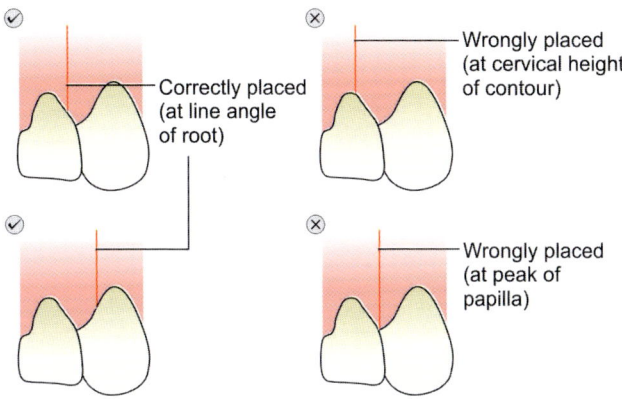

Fig. 4.57: Position of vertical incision

160. MODIFIED WIDMAN FLAP

Ramfjord and Nissle described the flap technique "Modified Widman flap."

Indications

- Pockets coronal to mucogingival junction.
- Sites where ostectomy surgery is not needed.

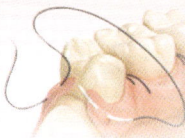

Contraindications

- Gingival overgrowth
- Bone deformities
- Inadequate zone of attached gingiva.

Technique (Figs 4.58A to M)

Step 1: Internal bevel incision (1st incision) is made 0.5 to 1 mm away from the gingival margin to the alveolar crest

Step 2: Flap reflection with periosteal elevator

Step 3: Crevicular incision (2nd incision) is made from the base of the pocket to the crest of the bone.

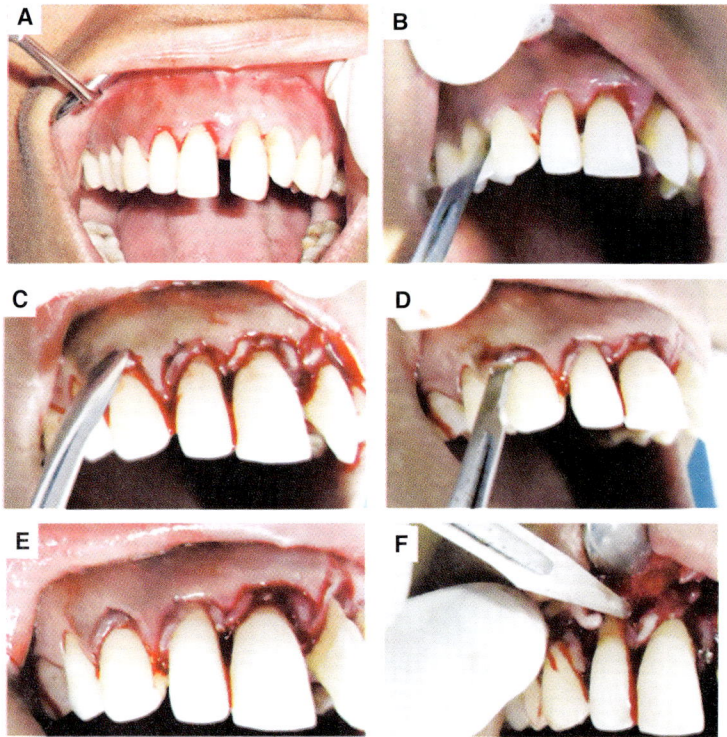

Fig. 4.58: Modified Widman flap: (A) Preoperative condition; (B) First incision; (C) Flap reflection; (D) Second incision; (E) First and second incision completed; (F) Third-interdental incision

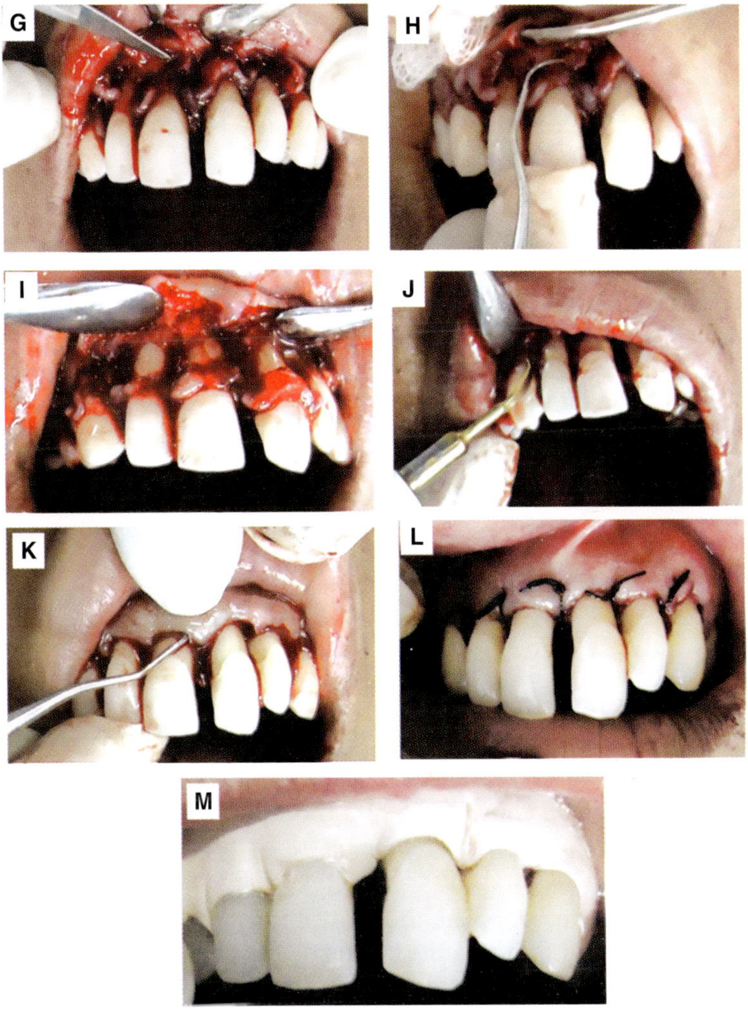

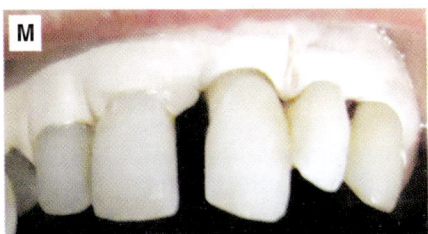

Fig. 4.58: Modified Widman flap: (G) Third incision contd; (H) Degranulation; (I) Removal of granulation tissue; (J) Removal of remnant of calculus; (K) Soft tissue thining; (L) Suturing; (M) Application of periodontal dressing

Step 4: Interdental incision (3rd incision) is made facially, lingually as well as interdentally, to free the gingiva completely around tooth.

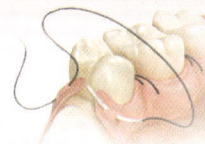

Step 5: Removal of triangular wedge-shaped granulation tissue. Degranulation and root planing.

Step 6: Proper adaptation of the interproximal tissue should be obtained by bone contouring wherever needed (osteoplasty) and thinning of the flap.

Step 7: Suturing of flap followed by periodontal dressing.

161. PAPILLA PRESERVATION FLAP

It was described by Takie in 1985.

Indications

1. Adequate interdental space
2. Esthetic zone
3. Reconstructive surgery.

Contraindication

1. Shallow vestibule
2. Tight or bodily contact of adjacent teeth.

Technique (Figs 4.59A to D)

Step 1: A crevicular incision around each tooth with no incisions across the interdental papilla.

Step 2: Semilunar palatal incision preserving interdental papilla. It should be 5 mm from the crest of the papilla so that the papilla can be incorporated into facial flap.

Step 3: Papilla is carefully dissected with Orban's knife.

Step 4: Dissected papilla is then elevated intact with facial flap; without thinning the tissue.

Step 5: Degranulation and reconstructive osseous surgery is performed, if indicated.

Step 6: Sutured and periodontal dressing given.

Advantages

1. Faster healing
2. Protection of grafted material.
3. Postoperative recession is less likely.
4. Better esthetic results.

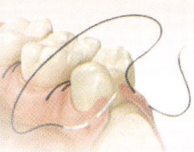

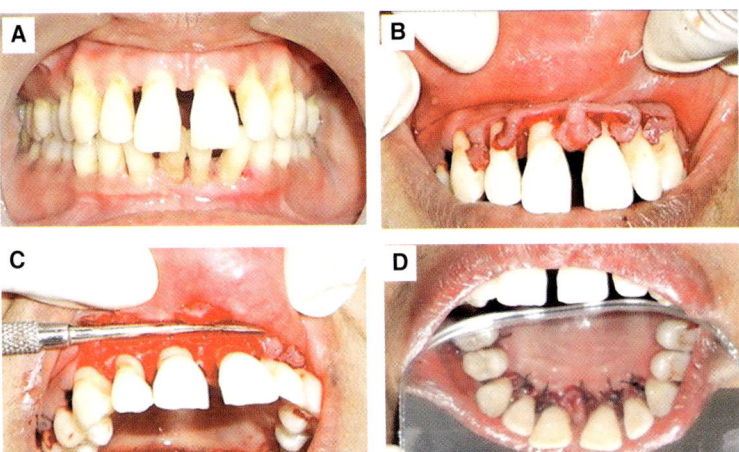

Fig. 4.59: Papilla preservation flap: (A) Preoperative condition; (B) Papilla preservation flap reflection; (C) Flap debridement; (D) Suturing

162. APICALLY DISPLACED OR POSITIONED FLAP

Indications

1. Widening the zone of attached gingiva.
2. Elimination of periodontal pocket.
3. Crown lengthening requiring ostectomy.

   Depending on purpose, it can be either split thickness or full thickness.

Contraindications

1. Deep infrabony defects.
2. Patient with high risk of caries.

Technique (Figs 4.60A to E)

Step 1: Internal bevel incision is made to preserve as much of keratinized and attached gingiva as possible. It is made 1 mm from the crest of gingiva directed to the bone.

Step 2: Crevicular incisions are made along with the flap reflection.

Step 3: Interdental incision and removal of wedge of granulation tissue.

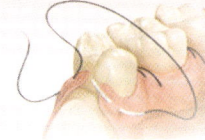

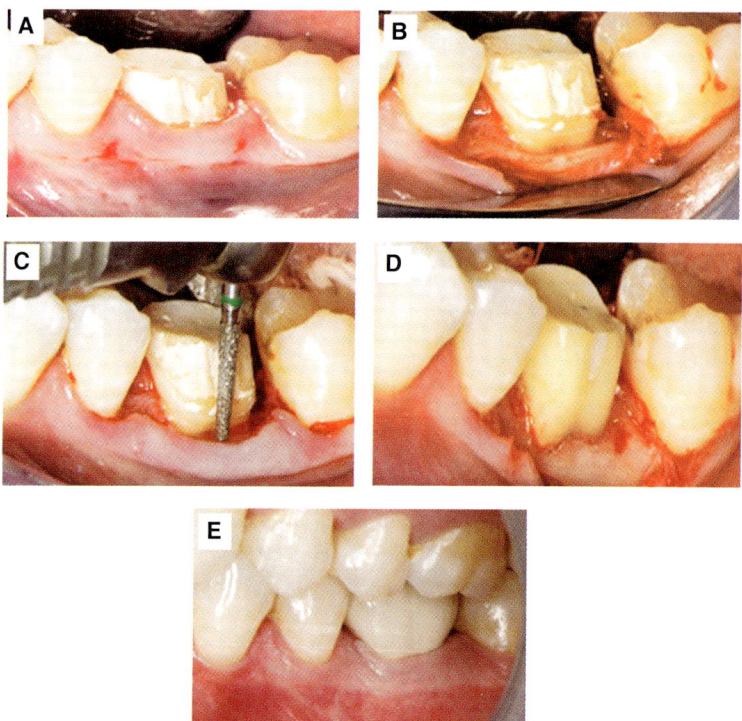

Fig. 4.60: Apically positioned flap: (A) Preoperative condition; (B) Flap reflection; (C) Osteoplasty; (D) After osteoplasty; (E) Postoperative condition

Step 4: Vertical incisions are made extending beyond the mucogingival junction to provide adequate mobility of flap to apical position.

Step 5: Root planing and degranulation

Step 6: Flap is sutured by sliding it apically on the bone.

Step 7: Periodontal dressing is applied which avoids the coronal shift of the flap.

Advantages

1. Eliminates the periodontal pocket.
2. Increases zone of attached gingiva.
3. Establishes gingival morphology facilitating good hygiene.

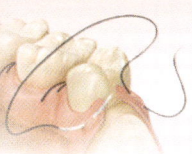

Disadvantages

Results in exposure of the roots causing esthetic problems and hypersensitivity.

163. CORONALLY POSITIONED FLAP

Indications

- Isolated gingival recession.
- Can be used with connective tissue grafting.

Contraindications

- Inadequate zone of attached gingiva.
- Deep recession defects
- Thin gingival biotype.

Basic Technique (Figs 4.61A to E)

Step 1: Vertical incisions on either sides extending beyond the mucogingival junction.

Step 2: Internal bevel incision from the gingival margin to the bottom of the pocket.

Step 3: Partial thickness flap or mucoperiosteal flap (as indicated) reflection with sharp dissection.

Step 4: Scaling and root planing.

Step 5: Place the flap and suture it at a level coronal to the pre-treatment position.

Step 6: Cover the area with periodontal dressing.

Variations of Coronally Positioned Flap

1. Semilunar coronally positioned flap (Tarnow) to cover denuded root surfaces.
2. Subepithelial connective tissue graft (Langer)
3. Pouch and tunnel technique.

Advantages

- Excellent color match
- Predictable root coverage

Disadvantages

- Cannot be done in deep recession defects.
- Semilunar CPF cannot be done for mandibular dentition.

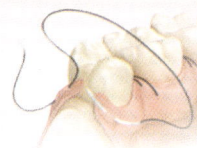

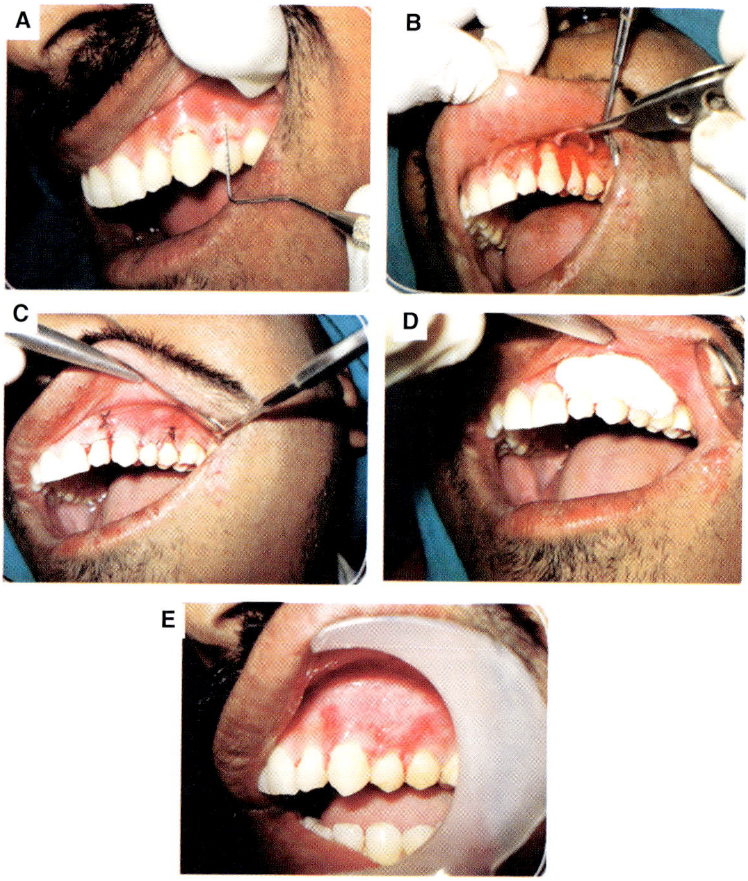

A **B**

C **D**

E

Fig. 4.61: Coronally positioned flap: (A) Preoperative codition; (B) Flap reflection; (C) Flap sutured coronally; (D) Periodontal dressing; (E) Post-operative condition

164. UNDISPLACED FLAP (INTERNAL BEVEL GINGIVECTOMY)

Indication

Gingival enlargement with periodontal pocket.

Technique (Fig. 4.62)

Step 1: Pockets are measured and marked with pocket marker and bleeding points are produced.

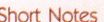
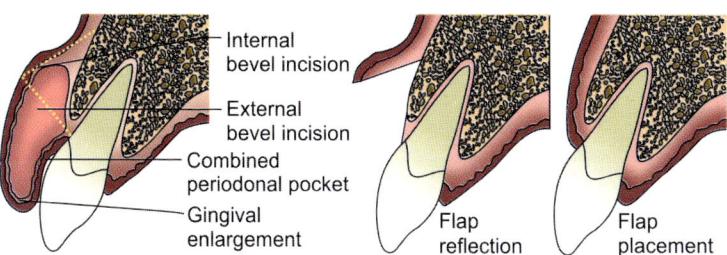

Internal
bevel incision

External
bevel incision

Combined
periodonal pocket

Gingival
enlargement

Flap
reflection

Flap
placement

Fig. 4.62: Undisplaced flap

Step 2: The internal bevel incision is made after the scalloping of the bleeding marks on the gingiva, pointing apical to the alveolar crest.

Step 3: Crevicular incision is made from base of the pocket to the bone to detach connective tissue.

Step 4: Flap reflection.

Step 5: The interdental incision is made with interdental knife, separating the connective tissue from bone.

Step 6: The triangular wedge is removed with a curette.

Step 7: Degranulation and root planing

Step 8: Trimming of the flap, if necessary, to allow the flap edge to end at the root bone junction.

Step 9: Suturing followed by periodontal dressing.

165. PALATAL FLAP

Palatal tissue is all attached, keratinized and lack the elastic properties. Therefore, it cannot be displaced or splited.

The initial incision for palatal flap should be such that, it should be precisely adapted at the root bone junction after suturing.

Flap should be thin to adapt to the underlying osseous tissue.

If the surgery is intended for debridement, the internal bevel incision is planned. While performing osseous surgery, the initial incision is located at lower level as per bone level.

The apical portion of the scalloping should be narrower than the line angle area because the palatal roots taper apically.

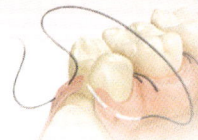

166. HEALING AFTER FLAP SURGERY

After suturing (up to 24 hours), a thin blood clot formed which connects the flap to underlying tooth or bone. It consists of fibrin reticulum with PMN leukocytes, erythrocytes, debris of injured cells and capillaries.

Few days (1 to 3) after flap surgery, the gap between flap and underlying tooth or bone becomes thinner with epithelial cell migration. There is inflammatory response to some extent.

An epithelial attachment to the root by means of hemidesmosomes and a basal lamina has been established after one week. The blood clot is replaced by granulation tissue.

After two weeks, collagen fibers begin to appear parallel to the tooth surface. Union of the flap to the tooth is still weak because of the presence of immature collagen fibers; although the clinical aspect may be normal.

It takes around one month for complete epithelized gingival crevice and a well-defined epithelial attachment to form. Functional arrangement of the supracrestal fibers begins to form.

Full thickness flap, which exposes the bone, results in superficial bone necrosis at initial few days, which declines thereafter. This results in some amount of bone loss.

After osteoplasty, the initial loss of both radicular and interdental bone follows bone repair in cancellous areas while marginal bone loss in relatively thin and unsupported cortical bone.

167. ROOT BIOMODIFICATION

Periodontal disease results in following changes in root surface wall of periodontal pocket.

1. Accumulation of bacteria and their products.
2. Degeneration of Sharpey's fibers.
3. Disintergration of cementum and dentin.

These changes interfere with new attachment. However, these changes can be eliminated either by thorough root planing and/or by treating the root surface by root conditioners. Application of certain substances for conditioning the root is

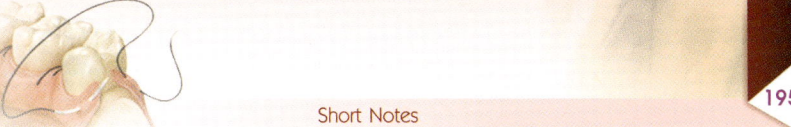

called root biomodification which improves the acceptance of new attachment.

Several substances have been proposed for this purpose.

1. Citric acid (pH of 1.0) applied on root surface and left for 2 to 5 minutes.
2. Fibronectin is a glycoprotein which is required for attachment of fibroblasts to the root surfaces. Application of fibronectin to the root surface may promote new attachment.

Tetracycline: Tetracycline, if applied on root surface, can improve new attachment by following ways.

a. Increases binding with fibronectin thereby stimulating fibroblast attachment.

b. Removes smear layer and exposes dentinal tubules.

Tetracycline has shown better results for connective tissue attachment.

168. CITRIC ACID IN ROOT SURFACE PREPARATION

Citric acid (pH 1), when applied for 2 to 3 minutes on root surface, produced a surface demineralization, induced cementogenesis and attachment of collagen fibers.

The actions of citric acid on root surfaces are as follows:

1. Citric acid induces accelerated healing and new cementum formation.
2. Citric acid has shown in vitro to eliminate endotoxins and bacteria from the diseased tooth surface.
3. Topically applied citric acid on periodontally diseased root surfaces, after root planing produces, a 4 micron deep demineralized zone with exposed collagen fibers.
4. Citric acid application not only removes the smear layer, exposing the dentinal tubules but also makes the tubule appear wider and with funnel-shaped orifices.
5. Epithelium does not migrate apically along denuded roots treated with citric acid. However, use of citric acid as root conditioner is controversial.

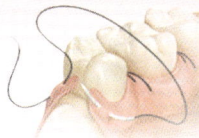

169. OSTEOPLASTY

Osteoplasty refers to reshaping of the bone without involving or removing the tooth supporting bone, i.e. the bone that does not provide attachment for periodontal ligament fibers. In this procedure, the existing bony topography is changed to eliminate periodontal pockets and this bony configuration allows the overlying gingiva to follow the contours of the underlying bone and establish shallow gingival sulci. As a result, patients have access for plaque control and can more effectively maintain the health of their own dentition and periodontium. The osteoplasty is performed to remove ledges, exostoses and tori (Figs 4.63A to D). It is used to reduce tuberosities, to give edentulous areas a saddle shape, and to establish grooves apical to the interdental spaces and furcations and distal to terminal teeth. Osteoplasty places the bone over the roots into facial and lingual prominences. This thinning of the alveolar housing narrows the buccal and lingual walls of interdental defects and thus facilitates their treatment. Surgical bone files, chisels and curettes are employed to eliminate interdental defects and to establish an ideal bony contour.

Fig. 4.63: Osteoplasty: (A) Preoperative condition; (B) Bony ledge; (C) Osteoplasty; (D) Postoperative condition

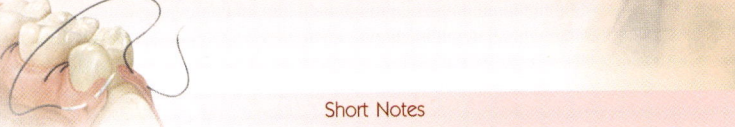

Osteoplasty includes the techniques of grooving or festooning and radicular blending to reduce the buccal and lingual thickness of bone interdentally.

170. BONE GRAFT MATERIALS

The goal of periodontal therapy is the reconstruction of the bone and ligamentous attachment that has been destroyed by disease. Several therapeutic methods may be used to reach this goal; one of these is bone grafting. The objective of bone grafting is the restoration of lost alveolar bone and the regeneration of a functional attachment.

A graft is a viable tissue that, after removal from a donor site, is implanted within a host tissue which is then restored, repaired or regenerated.

Points governing material selection (According to Schallorn):

1. Biologic acceptability
2. Predictability
3. Feasibility
4. Minimal operative hazard and postoperative sequelae
5. Patient acceptance

Bone graft is of following types:

a. An autograft is a bone transferred from one position to a new position in the same individual.

b. An allograft is a bone graft between individuals of the same species.

c. Xenograft is the bone graft between members of differing species.

d. Alloplast is an inert foreign body used for implantation in to tissue (non-bone material).

Bone graft materials are generally evaluated based on their osteogenic, osteoinductive or osteoconductive potential.

Graft Materials

1. **Autografts:** Cortical bone chips, osseous coagulum, bone blend, etc. It can be obtained either from extraoral or intraoral sites.

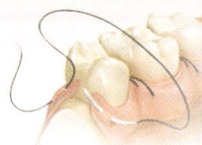

A. **Osseous coagulum:** It is mixture of bone dust and blood which is packed into the defect.

B. **Bone blend:** Uses an autoclaved plastic capsule and pestle in which bone removed from intraoral sites its triturated which is then packed into the defect.

C. **Bone swaging:** Bone is pushed into the defect from the adjacent edentulous area to contact the root surface without fracturing it at the base.

2. **Allografts:** Two types—freeze-dried bone allografts (FDBA) and decalcified freeze-dried bone allorgrafts (DFDBA).

3. **Xenografts:** Boplant (calf bone), Ospurum (cow bone), Boiled bovine bone, Kiel bone, Bio-oss (bovine derived).

4. **Alloplasts** (non-bone graft material): Sterile plaster of Paris, hydroxyapatite, calcium phosphate biomaterials.

171. GUIDED TISSUE REGENERATION (GTR)

To treat the periodontal disease, elimination of junctional and pocket epithelia may not be sufficient, because the epithelium from the excised margin may rapidly proliferate apically to become interposed between the healing connective tissue and the cementum. Several methods have been proposed to prevent or retard the migration of the epithelium. One of the methods is guided tissue regeneration. In this approach of prevention of epithelial migration along the cemental wall of the pocket consists of placing barriers of different types to cover the bone and periodontal ligament. Because only the periodontal ligament cells have the potential for regeneration of the attachment apparatus of the tooth and excluding the epithelium and the gingival connective tissue from the root surface during post-surgical phase favors repopulation of the areas by periodontal ligament and bone cells.

Two types of barrier membranes have been used.

1. Degradable (collagen, polyglactin, biobrane, periosteum) gets resorbed, do not require removals.

2. Non-degradable—requires removal after 3 to 6 weeks.

Non-degradable membranes, such as millipore filters, Teflon membranes, resulted in regeneration of cementum, alveolar bone and a functional periodontal ligament. Clinical studies have shown that GTR results in a gain in attachment level, but not necessarily with a buildup of alveolar bone.

The use of polytetrafluoroethylene (PTFE) membranes, Goretex periodontal membrane has been tested and has shown statistically significant decrease in pocket depths and improvement in attachment levels after 6 months.

172. ETIOLOGY AND CLASSIFICATION OF FURCATION INVOLVEMENT

Etiology of bifurcation and trifurcation involvement is microbial plaque.

1. The difficulty and sometime impossibility of controlling plaque in furca area is responsible for the presence of extensive lesions in the furcations.
2. Trauma from occlusion should be suspected as a contributing factor in cases of furcation involvement with crater-like or angular deformities in the bone.
3. Presence of enamel projections into the furca may play a role in initiation of furcations involvement.
4. The presence of accessory pulpal canals in the furcations area may extend pulpal inflammation to the furcation.

Classification of furcation involvement: The classification is based on horizontal type of bone loss or vertical type of bone loss.

1. Glickman's (horizontal) classification:

   Grade I: Incipient or early involvement of furcations with suprabony pockets and early interradicular bone loss. No radiographic changes (Fig. 4.64A).

   Grade II: Any involvement of the interradicular bone without through-and-through probability. Radiograph may or may not reveal this type of furcations (Fig. 4.64B) (cul-de-sac).

   Grade III: Through-and-through loss of interradicular bone. Mandibular molars may reveal radiolucency on radiograph (Fig. 4.64C). It is not visible clinically and filled with soft tissue.

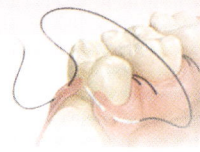

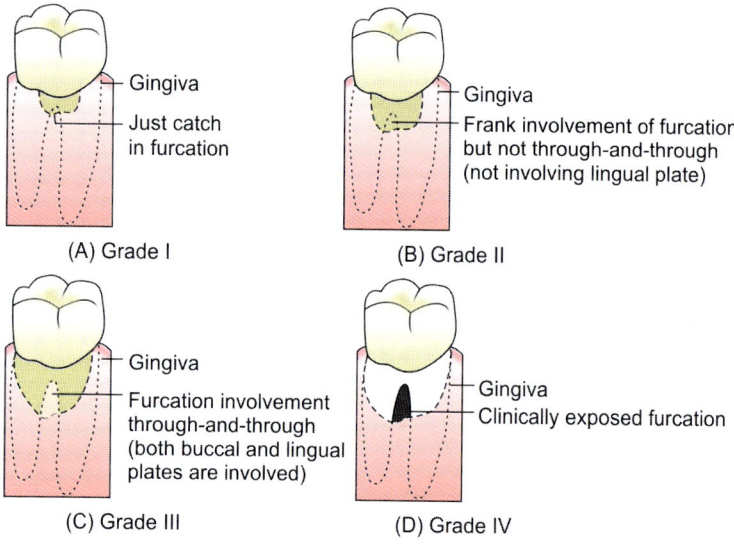

Fig. 4.64: Furcation involvement

Grade IV: Through-and-through loss of interradicular bone, with total exposure of furcations owing to gingival recession (Fig. 4.64D). It is visible clinically.

2. Tarnow and Fletcher (vertical) sub-classification: That measures the probeable vertical depth from the roof of the furca apically.

Grade A : Vertical loss of 1 to 3 mm.

Grade B : Vertical loss of 4 to 6 mm.

Grade C : Vertical loss of 7+ mm.

Furcation involvements can be best detected clinically by Naber's probe (Figs 4.65 and 4.66).

173. TREATMENT OF FURCATION INVOLVEMENT

Furcation lesions are treated by different therapeutic procedures depending on the severity of the involvement.

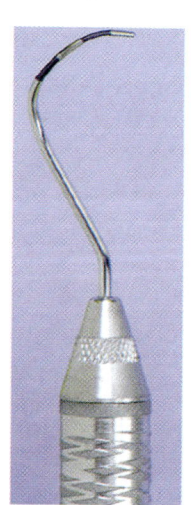

Fig. 4.65: Naber's probe

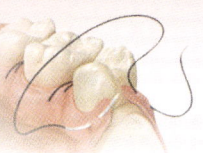

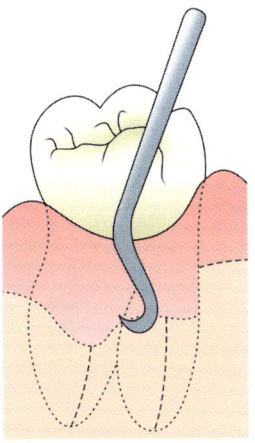

Fig. 4.66: Checking of furcation with Naber's probe

Treatment of grade I involvement: Usually suprabony pockets are present, which are treated by scaling and curettage or by gingivectomy depending on consistency of the pocket wall and depth of the pocket. In the early furcation involvements, and if the trauma from occlusion is the etiologic and aggravating factor, reshaping of the tooth (odontoplasty) is done.

Treatment of grade II involvement: Scaling and root planing of the teeth, with mucoperiosteal flap is done to treat the pathology which is usually present on one aspect or side of the tooth. Depending on the pattern of bone destruction within the interradicular area, bone grafting with or without guided tissue regeneration is performed.

Treatment of grade III and IV involvements: In these conditions, the interradicular tissue destruction permits a probe to pass freely through the furcations. The treatment is same as grade I and II. However, when infrabony pockets and osseous defects are present, bone contouring as well as instrumentation of the root surface facing the furcations, is required. The treatment of advanced grade II and grade III furcations involvement will often require the removal or resection of a root. This will allow access to the remaining root surfaces for scaling and root planing and for the patient's regimen of plaque control.

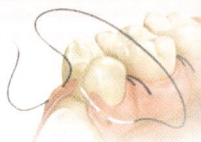

The treatment of advanced grade III and grade IV furcations involvement of mandibular molar can be accomplished by hemisection. Hemisection involves splitting of two rooted tooth in two separate portions (bicuspidization). After sectioning the tooth, one or both roots can be retained. In most of the cases of hemisections and root resections, the endodontic therapy is accomplished first (Figs 4.67A to F).

Extraction of the involved tooth may be indicated in cases of advanced attachment loss.

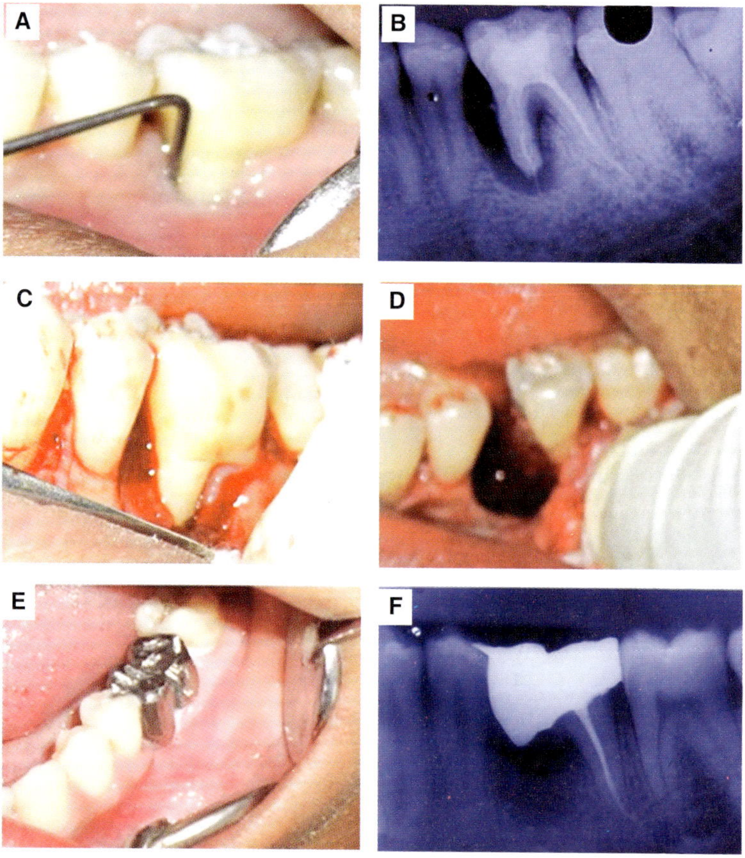

Fig. 4.67: Hemisection: (A) Preoperative mesial pocket; (B) Preoperative IOPA; (C) Flap reflection; (D) Mesial half of the tooth removed; (E) Restoration; (F) Postoperative IOPA

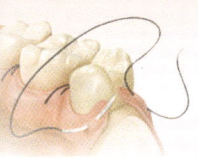

174. INDICATIONS FOR PERIODONTAL PLASTIC SURGERY (MUCOGINGIVAL SURGERY)

Periodontal plastic surgery consists of surgical procedures for the correction of gingiva–mucous membrane relationships that complicate periodontal disease and may interfere with the success of periodontal treatment.

Indications

1. To reposition the frenum.
2. To stop or prevent gaping of gingival or periodontal pockets caused by frenum pull. Tension from such attachments distends the gingival sulcus and fosters the accumulation of irritants that lead to gingivitis and pocket formation, and aggravates the progression of periodontal pockets and causes their recurrence after treatment.
3. It is indicated where the base of the periodontal pockets is apical or close to the mucogingival junction.
4. To increase the width of attached gingiva
5. To correct the esthetic problems.
6. Tissue engineering.

Often mucogingival surgery is performed in conjunction with procedures for correction of underlying osseous and anatomic deformities.

175. FREE GINGIVAL AUTOGRAFTS

Free gingival grafts (FGG) are used for widening the zone of attached gingiva and to cover denuded roots. There are various techniques of free gingival grafts: (1) The classic technique, (2) The accordion technique, (3) The strip technique, (4) The connective tissue technique and (5) Combination of strip and connective tissue technique.

The graft is initially maintained by a diffusion of fluid from the host bed, adjacent gingiva and alveolar mucosa. The fluid transudates from the host vessels and provides nutrition and hydration essential for the initial survival of the graft. Functional integration of the graft occurs by the seventeenth day and the graft will eventually blend with adjacent tissues.

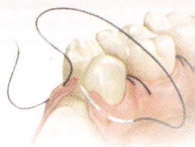

Miller modified the original classic technique of FGG to augment the gingiva coronal to recession. Modification includes root biomodification prior to preparation of recipient bed.

Classic Technique of Free Gingival Autograft (by Miller)
(Figs 4.68A to H)

Step 1: *Root planing and biomodification*

Step 2: *Preparation of recipient site*: To form a firm connective tissue bed to receive the graft. Horizontal incision is made followed by vertical incisions at the line angles of the adjacent teeth, tissue retracted and excised. Care should be taken to leave periosteum intact.

Step 3: *Obtain the graft from the donor site*: It consists of transferring a piece of keratinized gingiva of approximately the size of recipient site. Ideal thickness of the graft is between 1.0 and 1.5 mm.

Step 4: *Transfer and immobilization of graft*: The graft is positioned and adapted firmly to the recipient site. Then suturing of the graft is done without avoiding excessive tension. Minimal possible trauma to the graft yield better results.

Step 5: *Protect the donor site*: The donor site is covered with a pack for 1 week or more. Pack is retained by locking it interproximally or by a plastic stent wire or modified Hawley's retainer.

176. PEDICLE AUTOGRAFT (LATERALLY OR HORIZONTALLY SLIDING FLAP)

This technique of flap is used to cover facial root surface of individual tooth denuded by gingival recession.

Technique (By Grupe and Warren)

Step 1: *Preparation of recipient site*: Gingival margin is removed around the denuded root surface and then it is thoroughly scaled and planed.

Step 2: *Preparation of flap*: A full or partial thickness flap may be used. Vertical incision is given from the gingival margin to outline a flap adjacent to the recipient site

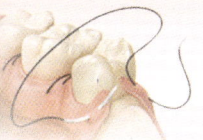

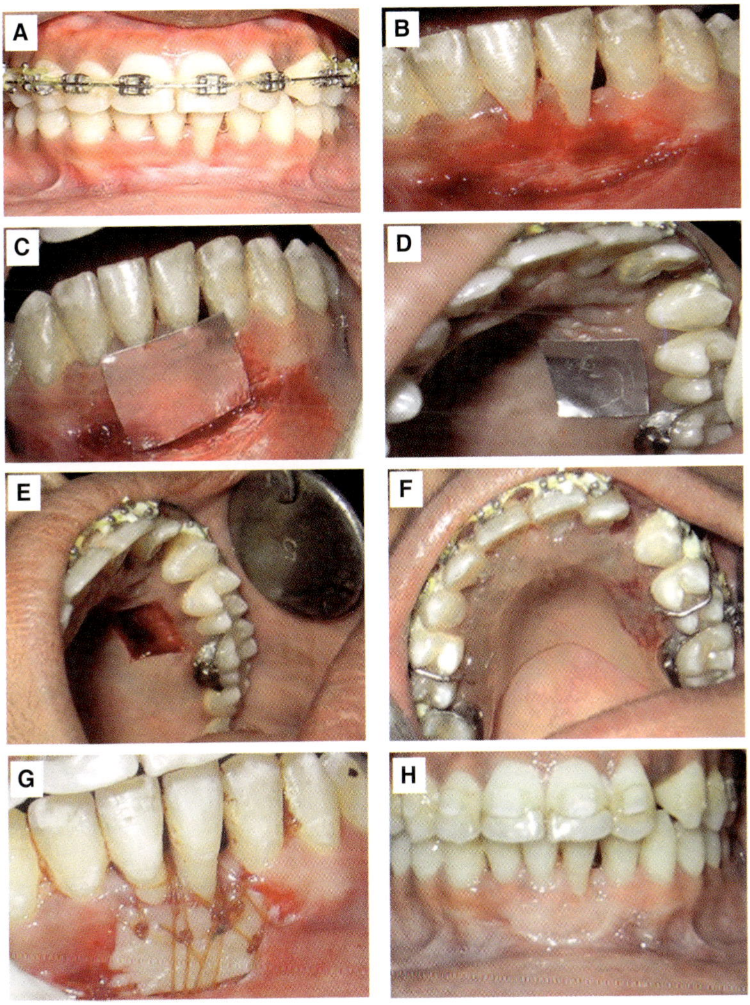

Fig. 4.68: Free gingival graft: (A) Preoperative condition; (B) Preparation of recipient bed; (C) Template; (D) Template at donor site; (E) Graft harvesting; (F) Protection of donor site; (G) Graft in place; (H) Post-operative condition

extending beyond the mucogingival junction. The flap should be sufficiently wider than the recipient site to cover the root. A partial thickness flap is reflected leaving the periosteum on the bone.

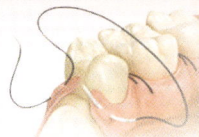

Step 3: *Flap transfer*: Slide the flap laterally to cover the recipient site. Suture the flap to adjacent gingival and the alveolar mucosa with interrupted sutures.

Step 4: *Protect the flap and donor site*: Cover the operative field with aluminum foil and a soft periodontal dressing.
- Remove the dressing and the sutures after one week.
- Varient techniques: Double papilla pedicle graft.
- Laterally moved coronally advanced flap.

177. CONNECTIVE TISSUE AUTOGRAFT

It was originally described by Edel.

Technique (Figs 4.69A to G)

Step 1: Divergent vertical incisions are made at the line angles of the tooth to be covered, creating a partial thickness flap to at least 5 mm apical to the receded area.

Step 2: Suture the apical mucosal border to the periosteum using resorbable suture.

Step 3: Thoroughly scale and plane the root surface simultaneously reducing the prominence.

Step 4: From the palate, a connective tissue graft is obtained and donor site is sutured after harvesting the graft.

Step 5: Transfer the graft to the recipient site and suture it to the periosteum with resorbable sutures. Good stability of the graft should be obtained with adequate sutures.

Step 6: Cover the grafted site with aluminum foil and periodontal dressing.

Advantages

1. Healing of donor site occurs by primary intention.
2. Less postoperative discomfort to the patient.
3. Better esthetics due to better color match.

178. TISSUE ENGINEERING

It is a non-invasive surgical procedure (Figs 4.70A to C). It has become a reality in recent years as a result of research and patient's demands.

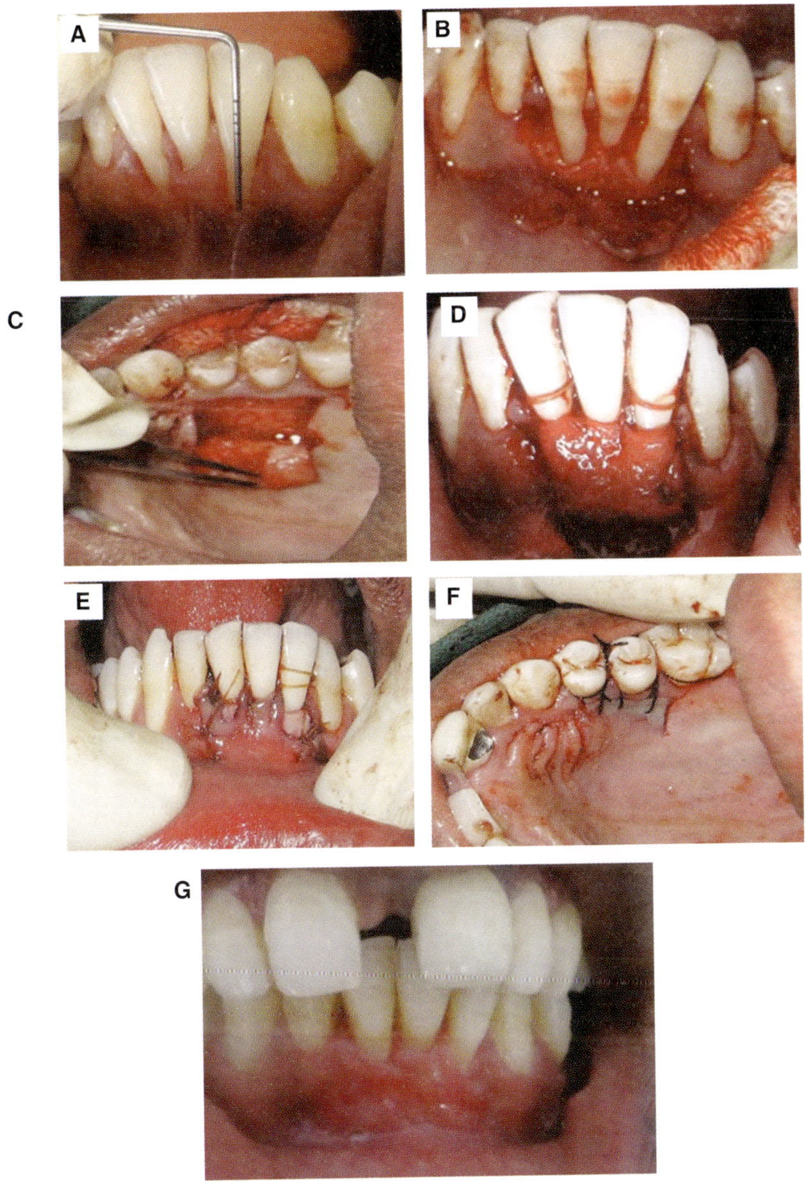

Fig. 4.69: Connective tissue autograft: (A) Preoperative condition; (B) Preparation of recipient bed; (C) Harvesting connective tissue graft; (D) Graft in place; (E) Suturing; (F) Donor site; (G) Postoperative condition

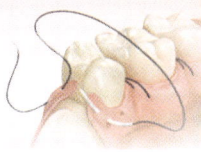

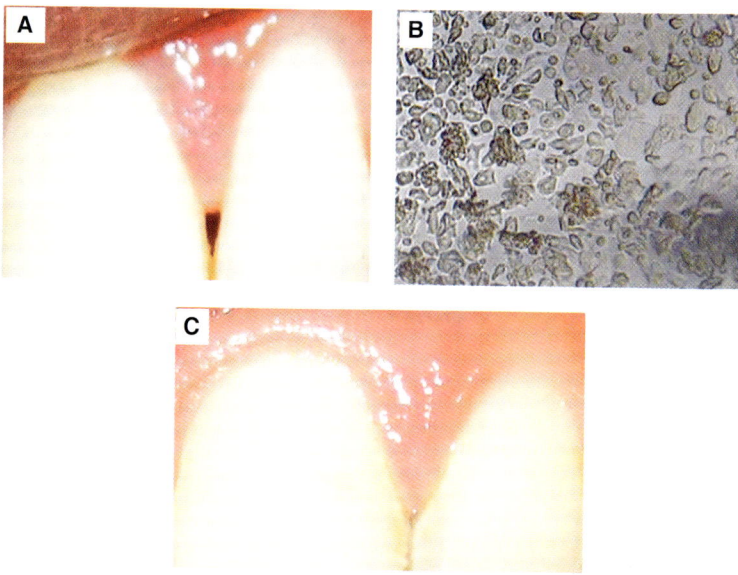

Fig. 4.70: Papilla regeneration by tissue engineering: (A) Short interdental papilla with un-esthetic black triangle; (B) Cultured gingival fibroblasts; (C) By injecting cultured gingival fibroblasts

Periodontal therapy has been involved with tissue engineering for many years, beginning with GTR that excluded certain cell types and created an engineered wound left to heal with appropriate cell types.

Tissue engineering based on materials used, is divided into passive and active categories to recognize the role the cells play.

Passive Engineering

1. Passive engineering: Therapies based on guided tissue regeneration
2. Biologically based acellular dermal matrix (ADM)

Active Engineering

1. Enamel matrix derivative (EMD)
2. Growth factors + beta tricalcium phosphate + collagen wound dressing.

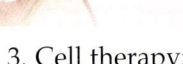

3. Cell therapy:
    a. Autologous fibroblast: Isolagen
    b. Bilayered cell therapy
    c. Dermagraft.

The reconstruction of the open interproximal space remains one of challenges in esthetic periodontal therapy. Autologous fibroblasts were injected into the interdental papilla in a method to atraumatically augment deficient gingival papilla.

Further studies are required for passive and active engineering for its validity on long-term basis.

179. SUPPORTIVE PERIODONTAL TREATMENT (SPT)

Patients are carried in the maintenance phase for a lifetime. Scientific evidence clearly shows that periodontal treatment can be successful in the vast majority of patients. One of the major elements of successful periodontal treatment is an effective maintenance programme.

Sequence of periodontal treatment phases:

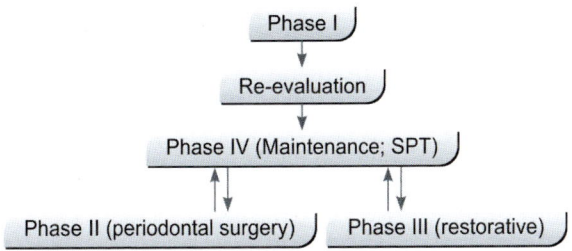

Maintenance Recall Procedures

Part I: Examination

- Medical history
- Oral examination
- Oral hygiene status
- Gingival, pocket depth and mobility changes
- Occlusal changes
- Dental caries
- Restorative and prosthetic phase.

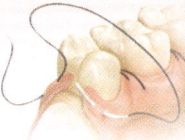

Part II: Treatment
- Oral hygiene reinforcement
- Scaling root planing and polishing
- Chemical irrigation

Part III: Report, clean up and scheduling
- Write report and discuss it with the patient.
- Clean and disinfect operatory.
- Schedule next recall visit
- Schedule further periodontal treatment.
- Schedule for prosthetic restorative treatment.

Recall interval: The interval between recall appointments must be tailored to each patient. For patients with excellent results— 6 months to 1 year; good results—3 to 4 months; and poor results—1 to 3 months.

During the recall visits, it is advisable to review the nature of the dental treatment the patient has previously received and the prognosis assigned to the dentition.

180. IMPLANT AND OSSEOINTEGRATION

Dental implant: Any material placed in jaw bone for the purpose of tooth replacement is called "Dental Implant". The best acceptable material for it is commercially available pure titanium. Implants can be either subperiosteal or endosseous. Endosseous implants are commonly used nowadays.

Types of endosseous implant:
- Blade, pin, disk, implants
- Root form implants

Implants can also be surface treated or non-surface treated.

Osseointegration: It is the formation of a direct stable interface between an implant and bone. Histologically osseointegration is the direct structural and functional connection between the surface of implant and surrounding bone without intervening soft tissues.

Clinically, it represents the rigid fixation or an implant in bone which can withstand the occlusal forces (Figs 4.71A to D).

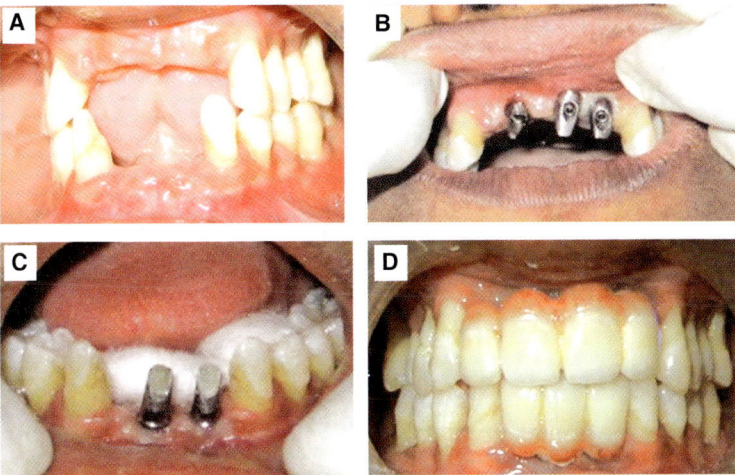

Fig. 4.71: Dental implants: (A) Preoperative; (B) Maxillary implants; (C) Mandibular implants; (D) Final prosthesis

181. PERI-IMPLANTITIS

It is the inflammation of the tissues around an osseointegrated functional implant resulting in loss of supporting bone.

It can be diagnosed by:

a. Careful probing with plastic probes
b. Radiographs
c. Clinical changes, such as suppuration, calculus, swelling, color change, bleeding and mobility.

Etiology

- Bacterial infection
- Immediate placement of implants after extractions
- Immediate loading after implant placement
- Screw loosening or fracture
- Fracture of implant or restoration.

Treatment

Peri-implantitis can be treated same as that of periodontitis; such as scaling, flap surgery with or without bone grafts or guided bone regeneration (GBR). Only thing that should be

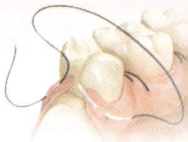

kept in mind that the instruments used for treatment of peri-implantits should be made up of plastic to avoid damage to the implant. In case of poor prognosis, the implants can be removed and eventually replaced.

182. LASERS IN PERIODONTICS

(LASER: Light Amplification by Stimulated Emission of Radiation.) Laser can concentrate light energy and exert a strong effect targeting tissue at an energy level much lower than natural light.

Different Types of Lasers

1. Neodymium: yttrium-aluminum garnet (Nd:YAG)—soft and hard tissue
2. Carbon dioxide (CO_2)—hard tissue
3. Diode laser—soft tissue
4. Erbium:YAG (Er:YAG)—soft and hard tissue
5. Argon: Soft tissue—limited use

Among these, high power lasers, such as CO_2, Nd:YAG, and diode lasers, can be used in periodontics.

Advantages:

1. Excellent soft tissue ablation.
2. Greater hemostasis
3. Bactericidal
4. Minimal wound contraction.

Disadvantage: Costlier

Precautions

1. Patient's and operator's eyes should be protected.
2. Proper irradiation technique and conditions need to be followed while using lasers.

Periodontal procedure's performed with lasers: In periodontics, the preferred laser is diode laser.

1. Gingivectomy and gingivoplasty.

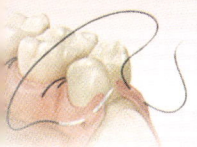

2. Crown lengthening
3. Depigmentation
4. Pocket sterilization
5. Excision of epulis
6. Use in implantology

183. PERIODONTAL MICROSURGERY

Microsurgery is aimed at improving surgical manipulations through better visual acuity and co-ordination. A surgical microscope or microsurgical loupes are used at magnification more than 10× which increases clinical accuracy.

In periodontics, microsurgical loupes and microscope can be successfully used for following procedures:

Root preparation: Magnification helps in creating clean and smooth root surface; which is the key factor in success of periodontal therapy.

Surgical periodontics: Specially indicated in aesthetically demanding periodontal plastic surgical procedures.

Advantages of periodontal microsurgery:
1. It allows less invasive surgical approach.
2. Less exposure of surrounding relatively healthy tissue as use of smaller surgical site.
3. Above two advantages enable less postoperative pain and rapid healing.
4. Butt joint wound created by microsurgery facilitates primary closure and enhances periodontal reconstructive possibility.
5. Microscopy permits easy identification of ragged wound edges for trimming and freshening.
6. Microsutures (6–0 to 9–0) can be efficiently used.

Microsurgical instruments: These are circular in cross-section to permit precise rotational movements. They are made up of titanium. It allows reduced unwanted hand movements thereby greatly reducing surgical fatigue.

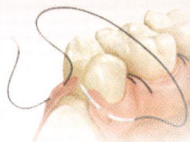

184. EVIDENCE-BASED DECISION MAKING (EBDM)

Evidence-based decision making rely on the best scientific evidences while making patient care decision.

Components of EBDM

1. Scientific evidence
2. Patient's preferences and values
3. Clinical patient circumstances
4. Experience and judgments.

To make the EBDM, only studies which have strong scientific base, properly controlled, unbiased, long term, not having commercial interest, with relevant hypothesis and properly randomized; are to be considered.

Example

A study of experimental gingivitis by Loe and co-workers has clearly shown that microbial plaque if not removed leads to gingivitis. When oral hygiene measures were instituted the gingivitis disappeared. This evidence clearly demonstrates that microbial plaque is the etiology of gingivitis.

185. DIAGNOSTIC INSTRUMENTS IN PERIODONTICS

1. Mouth Mirrors

Functions

- To provide indirect vision
- To retract lips, cheeks and tongue
- To reflect light

Characteristics

- **Flat surface mirrors:** Accurate and distortion free image
- **Concave mirrors:** Magnify images.
- **Double-sided mirrors:** Used to retract tongue or cheek and simultaneous view intraoral cavity.
- **Convex mirrors:** Cover large area although image is small.

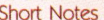
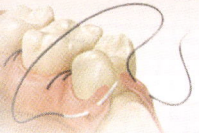

2. Explorers

Function

- To examine teeth for caries and calculus
- To check the smoothness after root planing.

Characteristics

- Pointed, sharp, thin but flexible tips
- Single- or double-ended.

Examples:

1. # 17 and 23
2. Pigtail
3. Orban's explorer
4. Shepherd's hook.

3. Cotton Forceps (Pliers or Tweezers)

Function

To grasp material or cotton and/or transfer it into and out of oral cavity.

4. Periodontal Probes

Function

- To measure the depth of the pocket
- To determine the configuration of the pocket.

Characteristics

Typical periodontal probe is tapered, rod-like with different calibrations and blunt rounded tip.

Examples

a. **Marquis color-coded probe:** Calibrations are in 3 mm sections.
b. **UNC-15 probe:** A millimeter markings at each millimeter and color-coding at the fifth, tenth and fifteenth millimeters.
c. **Michigan 'O' probe;** Markings at 3, 6 and 8 mm.
d. **University of Michigan 'O' probe with Williams marking:** Markings at 1, 2, 3, 5, 7, 8, 9 and 10 mm.
e. **WHO probe:** 0.5 mm ball at the tip and millimeter markings at 3.5, 8.5 and 11.5 mm and black band from 3.5 to 5.5 mm.

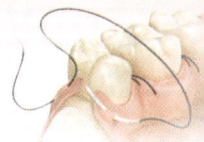

f. **Pressure sensitive probe:** Which has standardized, controlled insertion pressure.

g. **Naber's probe:** Used to detect furcation involvement.

186. FLORIDA PROBE

Conventional probing, although good and easy diagnostic method but is subjective and doesn't give a digital readout. To overcome these problems, an automated probe system was developed named as 'FLORIDA PROBE'.

Components

- Probe handpiece
- Digital readout
- Foot switch
- Computer interface
- Computer

Characteristics

- Diameter of end of the probe tip is 0.4 mm
- Measurements are done electronically and automatically transferred to computer when the foot switch is pressed.
- Constant probing force is provided.
- Objective readings.

Disadvantages

- Lack of tactile sensitivity.
- Constant force is applied regardless of the site of inflammation and may lead to inaccurate measurements and patients discomfort.

Other commercially available electronic probing systems are—interprobe and perioprobe.

187. PRINCIPLES OF PERIODONTAL INSTRUMENTATION

Effective instrumentation is governed by a number of general principles that are common to all periodontal instruments.

1. **Accessibility:** The position of the patient and operator should provide maximal accessibility to the area of operation. Every consideration should be given to patients comfort.

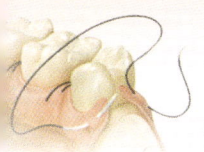

2. **Visibility, illumination and retraction:** Direct vision with direct illumination of dental light is most desirable. If this is not possible, indirect vision may be obtained by using the mouth mirror.

Retraction provides visibility, accessibility and illumination. The fingers and/or the mouth mirror are used for retraction.

3. **Condition of instruments:** Prior to any instrumentation, all instruments should be inspected to make sure that they are clean, sterile and in good condition. The working ends of pointed or bladed instruments must be sharp to be effective.

4. **Maintain a clean field:** Isolation of the area with cotton rolls, gauze pads and removal of blood and debris, aid in maintaining a clean operating field. As saliva interferes with visibility, adequate suction is essential and can be achieved with a saliva ejector or suction machine.

5. **Instrument stabilization:** Stability is essential for controlled action of the instrument and to avoid injury.

Two factors of importance in providing stability are the instrument grasp and the finger rest. The three methods for holding instruments in common usage are: (1) pen grasp, (2) modified pen grasp, and (3) palm and thumb grasp. The most effective and stable grasp for all periodontal instruments is the modified pen grasp.

6. **Finger rest:** The finger rest serves to stabilize the hand and the instrument by providing a firm fulcrum as movements are made to activate the instrument. Finger rest may be classified as intra- and extraoral finger rests. The intraoral finger rests are:

   1. Conventional   3. Opposite arch
   2. Cross-arch   4. Finger on finger.

   The two most commonly used extraoral fulcrums are:
   1. Palm-up
   2. Palm down.

7. **Instrument activation:** Correct angulation is must for effective calculus removal with precise adaptation to avoid injury to the soft tissue and with proper strokes.

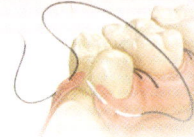

188. INSTRUMENTS USED IN PERIODONTAL SURGERY

1. **Cutting instruments (excisional and incisional):**
   - Periodontal knives
   - Surgical blades #12d,15,15c
   - Bard-Parker handle #3,4
   - Electrosurgery unit.
   - Laser unit

2. **Periosteal elevators:**
   - Glickman elevators
   - Woodson and Prichard elevators
   - Goldman Fox elevators

3. **Surgical curettes:**
   - Prichard curette
   - In addition, surgical hoes and files are also used.

4. **Surgical sickle:**
   - Ball scaler # B2-B3

5. **Surgical chisel:**
   - Ochsenbein paired chisels.

6. **Tissue forceps:**
   - DeBakey forceps

7. **Scissors:**
   - Goldman Fox scissors

8. **Needle holders:**
   - Conventional and Castroviejo needle holders.

9. **Suture materials:**
   - 3–0 or 4–0 mersilk
   - 3–0 chromic catgut
   - 3–0 vicryl
   - 5–0 vicryl or catgut for esthetic periodontal surgery.

10. **Insruments used for scaling and root planing:**
    Supra- and subgingival scalers
    - Manual
    - Ultrasonic

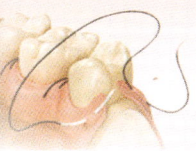

Supragingival scalers: Set. of 8

1. Interdental scalers (Jaquette scalers)
   a. Anterior interdental
   b. Pair of posterior interdental
2. Sickle scalers
   a. Large sickle for posteriors
   b. Small sickle for anteriors
3. Flat surface scalers
   a. Pair of flat surface scalers
   b. Cigulum/bifid scaler

Recently # UN 15–30 scaler is commonly used which is a combination of anterior interdental and large sickle scaler on either ends.

Subgingival scalers: Set. of 7

1. Hoe Scaler: Paired
2. Chiesel scaler of Zerfing's "Push" scaler
3. Root files—paired—restricted use.
4. Eyelet curette—paired
5. Universal and Gracey curretes.

All subgingival scalers are for both anteriors and posteriors.

11. Insruments used for osseous surgery:

1. Piezoelectric-surgical unit
2. Rongeurs   :   Friedman
              :   90° Blumenthal
3. Carbide round burs with slow speed handpiece.
4. Diamond burs
5. Interproximal files :   Schluger
                    :   Sugerman
6. Chisels: Backaction :   Ochsenbein Chisels.

189. ULTRASONICS IN PERIODONTICS

Ultrasonics are power-driven instruments used during periodontal therapy. These instruments work by converting

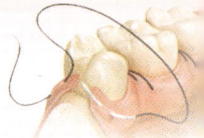

electric energy into mechanical energy in the form of high frequency vibrations of the instruments (18,000 – 50,000 cycles/ sec.) These vibratory actions cause fracture and dislodgement of the deposit from the tooth surface. A water lavage is continuously supplied to cool the tip and flush away the debris. Ultrasonic instruments are used for scaling and curettage.

Ultrasonics are of two types:

1. Magnetostrictive ultrasonic scalers
2. Piezoelectric ultrasonic scaler

Mechanism of Action

In ultrasonic scaler, detachment of calculus, microbial plaque and debris from tooth surfaces as well as from pockets is by following actions:

Acoustic streaming (flushing action) and automization: Water leaves the scaler forcefully thereby flushing the debris. At the tip of scaler, water comes out rapidly and in many directions, called as atomization.

Cavitation: Atomization leads to formation of local cavities in liquid as a result of decrease in total pressure. Cavitation is rapid formation and collapsing of bubbles creating vacuum in those places. When the bubble collapses, the phenomenon is called implosion; which causes release of enormous energy and pressure causing dislodgement of deposits from the tooth.

Acoustic turbulence: Ultrasonic waves cause disturbance in the flow of water causing acoustic turbulence. With continuous pressure produced within the confined space of the pocket, acoustic turbulence has the ability to mechanically remove dental calculus and bacterial plaque.

190. ORAL IRRIGATION

Oral irrigation effectively removes biofilm. For irrigation, continuous or pulsating stream of water or other solution is used. Pulsating oral irrigation device is more effective than continuous stream. Pulsation provides compression and decompression phases which result in clearing bacteria from periodontal pocket. It also allows control of pressure rate. These

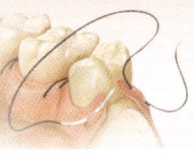

devices use 1200 pulsations per minute set on medium to high pressure settings (50–90 psi).

Oral irrigation devices create two zones: impact zone, in which the solution initially contacts and the flushing zone, in which solution enters into the subgingival area.

Oral irrigation can be supragingival or subgingival.

Supragingival irrigation is done with the jet tip placed above the gingival margin. Subgingival irrigation refers to the placement of soft, site-specific tip slightly below the gingival margin. Subgingival irrigation is indicated for the localized site, such as deep pocket, furcation or implant.

These devices use water or other solutions, such as diluted chlorhexidine or essential oils.

Home and in-office irrigation was found to be safe and effective in gingivitis, implants, orthodontics and periodontal maintenance.

191. CURETTES

Curettes are used for following purpose:

1. To remove subgingival calculus along with necrotic cementum.
2. To plane the root.
3. To remove the soft tissue lining of the periodontal pocket

Two basic types of curettes:

1. Universal: Designed for all areas
2. Area-specific curettes:
   - Gracey curettes
   - Extended shank curettes
   - Mini-bladed curettes
   - Langer and mini-Langer curettes

Universal curettes: One curette is designed for all areas and surfaces. It has cutting edges on both the sides.

Gracey curettes: These are area-specific curettes numbered from 1 to 14. Gracey curettes 11–12 and 13–14 are modified to 15–16 and 17–18.

Extended shank curettes (after 5 curettes): The shank is extended 3 mm than the standard Gracey curettes which allows

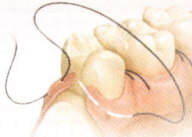

extension into deeper periodontal pockets. These are available in all Gracey numbers except 9–10.

Mini-bladed curettes (mini 5 curettes): These are modified area-specific curettes with the blade length half of that of the standard curettes. The shorter blade allows easier insertion, adaptation in deep narrow pockets as well as in furcation areas.
• Available in all standard Gracey numbers except 9–10.

Gracey curvettes: These are four mini-bladed curettes with the blade curved slightly upward; which allows the curette to adapt more closely to tooth surface and on line angles.

Sub-0 and 1–2—for anterior and premolars. 11–12—for posterior mesial surface. 13–14—for posterior distal surface.

Langer and mini-Langer curettes:

• This is set of 3 curettes.
• These have the shank designs of 5–6, 11–12 and 13–14 of Gracey's curettes with a universal blade.
• This modification permits advantage of both area-specific and universal curettes.
• Langer 1–2—mesial and distal of mandibular posteriors
• Langer 3–4—mesial and distal of maxillary posteriors.
• Langer 5–6—mesial and distal of anterior teeth

192. PERIODONTAL KNIVES

These are broadly categorized in two types:
1. Disposable scalpel blades.
2. Reusable periodontal knives:
   • Flat-bladed
   • Interproximal

Disposable scalpel blades: Surgical blades are available in market which can be mounted on BP handle and can be replaced.

Example: 12D, 15, 15C.

Flat-bladed knives: These are usually used for gingivectomy purpose hence called gingivectomy knives. These knives have broad and flat blades.

Example: Kirkland knife.

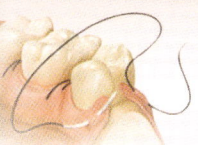

Interproximal knives: These have two long straight cutting edges that come together at the sharply pointed tip.

Example: Orban's knife.

Following are the important periodontal knives:
1. Goldman fox – Flat (GF #7)
   – Interproximal GF 8, 9, 11
2. Kirkland – Flat 15 K and 16 K
3. Orban – Interproximal — # 1 – 2
4. Merrifield – Interproximal — # 1, 2, 3, 4
5. Buck – Flat—# 3 – 4, 5 – 6
6. Sanders – Interproximal — # 1 and 2

193. SHARPENING OF PERIODONTAL INSTRUMENTS

Instruments must be sharp for effective scaling and root planing. Dull instruments not only increase working time and physical effort but also can burnish the calculus rather than remove it and cause tissue trauma as well.

Instrument sharpening is done with stones. Sharpening stones are available in various grits, designs and textures. Stones may be mounted or unmounted. Natural abrasive stones—India and Arkansas. Synthetically produced stone—Carborundum, Ruby and Ceramic stones (Fig. 4.72).

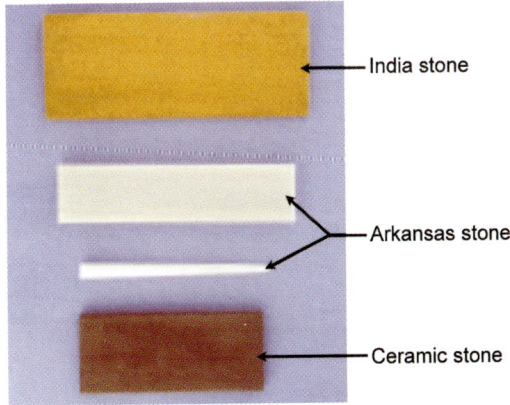

Fig. 4.72: Sharpening stones

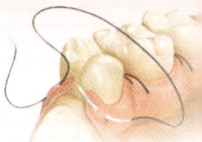

Objective of sharpening: To restore fine, thin, linear cutting edge of the instrument without distorting the original angles of it.

Evaluation of Sharpening

1. By sight: When a dull instrument is held under the light, the rounded surface of the cutting edge reflects light back to the observer. The acutely angled cutting edge of sharp instrument has no surface area to reflect light in contrast with the dull edge.

2. By touch: It is done by drawing the instrument lightly across an acrylic rod known as sharpening "test stick". A dull instrument will slide smoothly, without biting into the surface and raising a light shaving as a sharp instrument would do.

Principles of Instrument Sharpening

1. Instrument should be sharpened at the first sign of dullness. Proper size and shape stone or stones are used to avoid damaging the working end.

2. Entire cutting edge is ground evenly to avoid creating a new bevel at the cutting edge.

3. Surface of the sharpening stone must always be lubricated with a thin layer of lubricant (oil for natural and water for synthetic stones) during sharpening. Light but firm pressure is used. Excessive pressure, which generates heat and reduces control, should be avoided.

4. A firm, stable grasp of both the instrument and sharpening stone should be maintained to ensure proper angulation throughout.

5. A sterilized sharpening stone should be used.

6. Avoid formation of a "wire-edge".

The flat, unmounted hard Arkansas stone is the stone of choice for sharpening all instruments with straight cutting edges.

Honing the instruments: During sharpening process, bits of ground metal may remain attached to the edge of the instrument and creates a "wire-edge". As a final step in

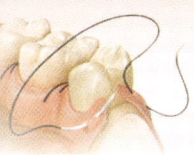

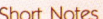

sharpening, this wire-edge should be removed by a process called honing. Honing is done with a flat Arkansas stone. The stone is moved gently and lightly along the entire non-beveled side of the cutting edge to obtain a finished edge.

194. SUTURING MATERIALS

Sutures are placed after periodontal surgery to maintain the flap in desired position until the primary healing has occurred.

For suturing, different types of suturing materials and suture needles are used in periodontal surgeries.

Suture materials: These are broadly classified as resorbable and non-resorbable. Both of these are further subdivided into monofilament or braided.

Most commonly used suture materials are:

Non-Resorbable

a. 3-0 Braided silk (natural)

b. 3-0 Ethicon, synthetic, monofilament.

Resorbable

Natural

a. Cat gut (3-0, 4-0, 5-0)

b. Chromic cat gut (3-0, 4-0, 5-0)

Synthetic

Vicryl

Resorbable sutures are preferred on non-resorbable because they enhance patient comfort and eliminate suture removal appointments.

Monofilament sutures are preferred over braided ones as it alleviates wicking effect of braided sutures thereby preventing the entry of bacteria to the deeper tissues from oral cavity.

195. PERIODONTAL DRESSINGS

Periodontal dressings are used to cover and protect wound surfaces after surgery. They have no curative properties, but protect the tissues thereby assist in healing. The primary

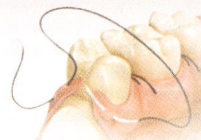

qualities of an ideal periodontal dressing are ability to immobilize and adopt the soft tissue to the tooth and underlying bone, reducing pain, preventing regrowth of tissue, reducing hemorrhage and postoperative infection, mechanical trauma and act as stent for mobile teeth. The dressing should also be comfortable and antimicrobial in nature.

Several types of dressings are available:

1. Zinc Oxide–Eugenol Dressings

Wondr–pak: Supplied as liquid and powder.

Advantages

i. Economic

ii. Good shelf life.

Disadvantages

i. Allergic reaction that produces reddening of the area and burning pain.

ii. Taste—incompatible to patient.

2. Non-Eugenol Dressing

A. **Coe-pak: Supplied in two tubes:** One tube contains—zinc oxide, oil (for plasticity), gum (for cohesiveness), Lorothidol (fungicide).

   Other tube contains—liquid coconut fatty acids, colophony rosin, chlorothymol (bacteriostatic agent).

B. **Other examples:**
   i. Cyanoacrylates
   ii. Tissue conditioners (methacrylate gels)
   iii. Periodontal varnish

Antibacterial properties of packs: Antibiotics like bacitracin, oxytetracycline, neomycin and nitrofurazone and antiseptics are adde)d in periodontal dressings to enhance wound healing.

Retention of packs: In an attempt to increase dressing retention, several techniques and materials have been suggested. These include stainless steel wire, dental floss, adhesive tin foil, self-cure acrylic, copper bands, stents, etc.

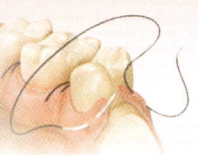

196. CLASSIFICATION OF PERIODONTAL INSTRUMENTS

Periodontal instruments

Diagnostic
- Mouth mirror
- Periodontal probes
- Explorer
- Tissue holder

Scalers

Supra-gingival
- Jacuettes
- Sickles
- Flat surface

Sub-gingival
- Hoe
- Chisel
- Curettes

Polishing
- Rubber cup
- Polishing brush
- Handpiece

Surgical
- Periodontal knives
- Surgical blades
- Periosteal elevators
- Bone files
- Rongeurs
- Scissors
- Needle holders

Miscellaneous
- Ultrasonic scalers
- Laser
- Diamond and carbide burs

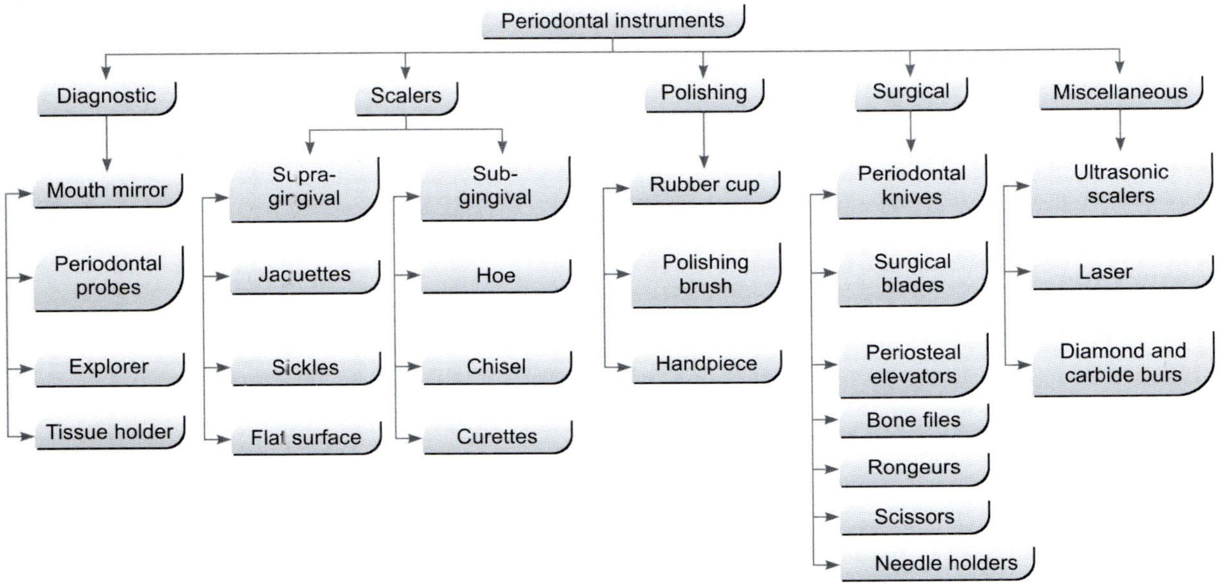

POINTS TO PONDER

1. Swallowing occurs approximately **600** times in 24 hours.
2. Total time of tooth contact in chewing and swallowing in 24 hours is **17.5 minutes** (approximately)
3. Thickness of oral epithelium: **0.2 to 0.3 mm**
4. Length of junctional epithelium—ranges from **0.25** to **1.35 mm**
5. Number of cellular layers of junctional epithelium—**10 to 29 cells** wide.
6. Free gingival groove—shallow linear depression between marginal and attached gingiva—about **1 mm** wide.
7. Width of attached gingiva
   a. Maxilla—Anterior—**3.5 to 4.5 mm**
   b. Mandible—Anterior—**3.3 to 3.9 mm**
   c. Least in mandibular first premolar—**1.8 mm**
8. Over jet and over bite—**0 to 2 mm**
9. Thickness of periodontal ligament—**0.13 to 0.21 mm**
10. Shape of periodontal ligament—**Hourglass**-shaped
11. Freeway space—Average **1.7 mm**
12. Biologic width—Average **2 mm**
13. Daily salivary secretion—**1 to 1.5 litres**
14. Diameter of toothbrush bristle – Ranges from **0.2** mm to **0.4 mm**
15. Toothbrush to be replaced—**Every 3 to 4 months**.
16. Thickness of cementum—**16 to 60 μm** to **150 to 200 μm** (equals to thickness of a hair)
17. Gingival sulcus depth **0 to 3 mm**
18. Distance from cementoenamel junction to alveolar crest—Average **1.08 mm** may increase up to **2.81 mm**
19. Predominant type of collagen in periodontium—**Type I**
20. Type of collagen in basal lamina—**Type IV**
21. Turnover time of gingiva—**10 to 12 days**
22. Turnover time of junctional epithelium—**1 to 6 days**
23. What is the relative volume of PMN in junctional epithelium after which the tissue looses cohesiveness and detaches from the tooth surface?— **60% or more**

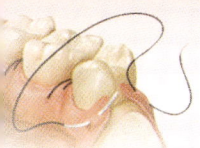

24. Rate of yearly bone loss in aggressive periodontitis—**0.1 to 1.0 mm**

25. Rate of yearly bone loss in chronic moderate periodontitis—**0.05 to 0.5 mm**

26. Rate of yearly bone loss in mild periodontitis—less than **0.05 mm**

27. Approximate number of bacteria present in one gram of plaque (wet weight)—**10^{11}**

28. Number of bacteria in healthy crevice—approximately—**10^3**

29. Approximate number of microbial species—**500**.

30. Radius of action: Bacterial plaque can induce bone loss within **1.5 to 2.5 mm** range of effectiveness. (According to Wearhaug)

31. What is wrong? What has happened?—**Diagnosis**

32. How did it happen?—**Etiology**

33. What can be done?—**Treatment**

34. What is going to happen?—**Prognosis**

35. How it can be prevented—**Prophylaxis**

36. By age 40, Physiologic mesial migration results in reduction of about **0.5 cm** in the length of the dental arch from midline to the third molar.

37. The body contains 10 times more bacteria than human cells.

38. The bacterial population comprises of 2 kg of the total body weight.

39. Corncob arrangement: It is a co-aggregation form of bacterial arrangement in which central core of gram-negative filamentous bacteria supports the outer coccal cells which are firmly attached.

40. Nicotine uptake of 34 g smokeless tobacco equals to 1.5 packs of cigarettes (approximately).

CASE HISTORY PROFORMA

Name   :   Case No.   :

Age   :   Date   :

Sex   :   Phone No. :

Occupation   :

Address   :

Chief Complaint :

History of Present Illness :

Past Dental History :

Medical History :

Oral Hygiene Procedures :

Any adverse habits :

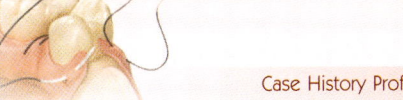

Extraoral Examination

➢ Face :

➢ Lymph nodes :

➢ Examination of temporomandibular joint (TMJ) :

➢ Any other :

Intraoral Examination

Gingival Status

   1. Color :

   2. Contour :

   3. Consistency :

   4. Size:

   5. Surface texture:

   6. Position of gingiva:

7	6	5	4	3	2	1	1	2	3	4	5	6	7

   7. Bleeding score:

   8. Suppuration :

   9. Tension test :

  10. Width of attached gingiva :

     Anterior : Adequate/Inadequate

     Posterior : Adequate/Inadequate

  11. Others :

Hard Tissue Examination

1. Teeth present :

2. Missing :

3. Caries :

4. Wasting diseases of teeth :

5. Sensitivity :

6. Pain on percussion :

7. Occlusion : Traumatic/Atraumatic

8. Pathologic migration :

❖ OHI-S Index (Greene and Vermillion)

Tooth	Debris and Stains – Facial	Calculus – Facial	Tooth	Debris and stains – Oral	Calculus – Oral
16			36		
11					
26			46		
31					

Debris Index Score: $\dfrac{\text{(Total debris score)}}{6}$ =

Calculus Index Score: (Total calculus score/6) =

OHI-S Score: Debris index score + calculus index score
(0 – 0.6 Good; 0.7 – 1.8 Fair; 1.9 – 3.0 Poor)

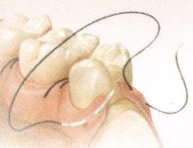

- Plaque Index (Turesky-Gilmore-Glickman modification of Quigley and Hein Index)

	17	16	15	14	13	12	11	21	22	23	24	25	26	27
F														
P														

	47	46	45	44	43	42	41	31	32	33	34	35	36	37
F														
L														

Plaque Score :

Periodontal Status :

(0 – 1.2 Good; 1.3 – 3.0 Fair; 3.1 – 6.0 Poor)

PROBING POCKET DEPTH: (Type of pocket- _____)

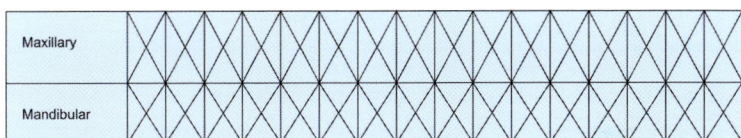

Provisional Diagnosis :

Investigations :

Final Diagnosis :

Prognosis :

– Overall prognosis

– Individual tooth prognosis

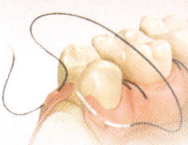

Treatment Plan :

- ➢ Emergency Phase

- ➢ Etiotropic Phase

- ➢ Surgical Phase

- ➢ Restorative Phase

- ➢ Maintenance Phase

BIBLIOGRAPHY

1. Carranza FA, Newmann MG: Clinical Periodontology, 8th edition; Sounders, 1996.

2. Glickman Irving: Clinical Periodontology, 3rd edition; Sounders, 1965.

3. Goldman HM, Cohen DW: Periodontal Therapy, 6th edition; Mosby, 1980.

4. Grant, Stern, Everett: Periodontics, 5th edition; Mosby, 1979.

5. Hoag PM, Pawlak EA: Essentials of Periodontics, 4th edition; Mosby, 1990.

6. Newman MG, Takei HH, Carranza FA: Clinical Periodontology, 9th edition; Saunders, 2003.

7. Newman MG, Takei HH, Carranza FA: Clinical Periodontology, 10th edition; Saunders, 2007.

5. Newman MG, Takei HH, Carranza FA: Clinical Periodontology, 11th edition; Saunders, 2012.

SECTION – B

(10 × 3 = 30)

❑ **Brief answer questions:**

   a. What are the pathways of spread of inflammation to the deeper periodontal structures?

   b. Define gingivectomy and mention the various methods of performing gingivectomy.

   c. Discuss the etiology of periodontal abscess.

   d. What is GTR?

   e. Define and classify dental plaque.

   f. What are the theories of calculus formation?

   g. What is fenestration and dehiscence?

   h. Mention the age changes in gingiva.

   i. What are the effects of smoking on periodontium?

   j. Define mucogingival surgery and give its indications.

SECTION – C

(2 × 10 = 20)

❑ **Long answer questions:**

   a. Define periodontal ligament and give its function.

   b. Define periodontal flap and discuss in details modified Widman flap.

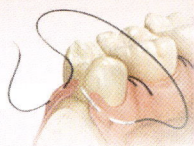

2   PATTERN PAPER

SECTION – B

(10 × 3 = 30)

❑ **Answer the following:**

  a. Steps of osseous resective surgery

  b. Uses and disadvantages of chlorhexidine.

  c. Specific and non-specific plaque hypothesis.

  d. Drug induced gingival enlargement.

  e. Comparison between Universal and Gracey curettes.

  f. Halitosis

  g. Gingival crevicular fluid

  h. Types of bone loss in periodontal diseases.

  i. Diabetes mellitus and periodontal diseases.

  j. Theories of mineralization of calculus.

SECTION – C

(2 × 10 = 20)

❑ **Long answer questions:**

  a. Define trauma from occlusion. Classify it with examples. Explain the role of TFO in causation of periodontitis.

  b. Define flap. Classify flaps. Describe modified Widman flap surgery.

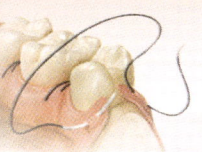
PATTERN PAPER   3

SECTION – B

(10 × 2 = 20)

❑ **Short answer questions:**
a. Functional of periodontal ligaments.
b. Classification of gingival recession.
c. Clinical features of desquamative gingivitis.
d. Local drug delivery.
e. Interdental cleansing Aids.
f. Coronoplasty.
g. Epulis
h. Supportive periodontal treatment.
i. Stress and periodontal disease.
j. Treatment of acute pericoronitis.

SECTION – C

(2 × 10 = 20)

❑ **Long answer questions:**
a. What is the rational of periodontal therapy? Describe in details the general principles of periodontal therapy.
b. What is prognosis? Enumerate various factors for determination of overall and individual prognosis. Discuss in detail individual prognosis in periodontitis case.

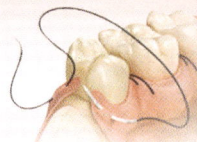

4   PATTERN PAPER

SECTION – B

(10 × 2 = 20)

❑ **Short answer questions:**

   a. Functional of periodontal ligaments.

   b. Periodontal pack.

   c. Local drug delivery.

   d. Crown lengthening surgery.

   e. Classify flaps

   f. Define and classify dental plaque.

   g. Guided tissue regeneration

   h. Chemical plaque control.

   i. Gingival curettage.

   j. Sharpening of periodontal instruments.

SECTION – C

(2 × 10 = 20)

❑ **Write long answer:**

   a. Classify gingival enlargement. Write a note on drug-induced gingival enlargement.

   b. Define furcation involvement. Describe the classification, clinical and radiographic features and treatment of furcation involvement.

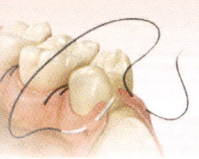
PATTERN PAPER 5

SECTION – B

(10 × 2 = 20)

❏ **Answer the following:**

a. Composition of dental plaque.

b. Stages of gingivitis.

c. Osseous craters.

d. Fenestration and dehiscence.

e. Individual tooth prognosis.

f. Disclosing agent.

g. Classification of flap.

h. Periodontal menefestation of HIV patient.

i. Pregnancy tumour.

j. Non-bone graft material.

SECTION – C

(2 × 10 = 20)

❏ **Write long answer:**

a. Enumerate acute gingival infections. Describe in details synonyms.

b. State the systemic condition in modifying the clinical appearance of periodontal tissue and describe in detail "Two-way relationship between diabetes mellitus and periodontitis.

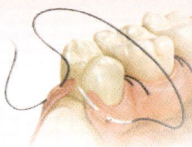

6   PATTERN PAPER

SECTION – B

(10 × 2 = 20)

❏ **Answer the following:**

a. Clinical features of acute necrotizing ulcerative gingivitis.

b. Periosteum and endosteum.

c. Risk factors for periodontal disease.

d. Oral malodours—extraoral causes.

e. Autogenous bone grafts

f. Biomodification of root surfaces.

g. Occlusion end periodontal health.

h. Chemical plaque control.

i. Classification with short description of periodontal pockets.

j. Mode of action of pathogenic microorganisms in periodontal diseases.

SECTION – C

(2 × 10 = 20)

❏ **Write long answer:**

a. Define periodontal plastic surgery.

- Present P.D. Millers classification of gingival recession diagrammatically.

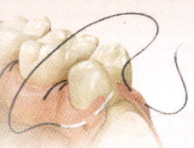
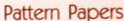
- Enumerate the techniques to increase the attached gingiva coronal to recession.
- Describe the free gingival autograft technique in short

b. Classify periodontal instruments.

- What are the principles of instrumentation?
- What are the different types of strokes used in periodontal instrumentation?

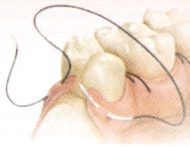

7   PATTERN PAPER

SECTION – B

(10 × 2 = 20)

❏ **Answer the following:**

   a. Idiopathic gingival enlargement.

   b. Guided tissue regeneration.

   c. Lamina dura.

   d. Iatrogenic factors

   e. Periodontal disease in diabetes.

   f. Leukocytes in dentogingival area.

   g. Anatomic factors in individual tooth prognosis.

   h. Healing after periodontal surgery.

   i. Treatment of acute pericoronitis.

   j. Oral irrigation.

SECTION – C

(2 × 10 = 20)

❏ **Write long answer:**

   a. Classify periodontitis. Describe the clinical and radiographic features and treatment of aggressive periodontitis in detail.

   b. Write in detail of the available classifications of gingival recessions for their merits and short comings.
     Enumerate the techniques described to achieve coronal augmentation of gingival recession with their merits and demerits. Describe any one technique in detail.

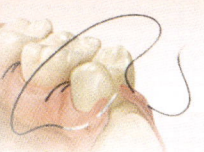
PATTERN PAPER   8

SECTION – B

(10 × 2 = 20)

❑ **Answer the following:**

a. Differentiate between attached gingiva and alveolar mucosa.

b. Describe the theories of calculus mineralization.

c. Define "trauma from occlusion" and describe the Tissue response to occlusal forces.

d. Define flap. Explain the incisions in modified Widman flap procedure.

e. Describe the micropography of the gingival wall of the periodontal pocket.

f. Explain the implant bone interface.

g. What is osseous coagulum?

h. Principles of sharpening of instruments.

i. Pregnancy tumour.

j. Define gingivectomy and explain the procedure.

SECTION – C

(2 × 10 = 20)

❑ **Write long answer:**

a. Define furcation involvement. What are the grades of furcation involvement? Describe in detail the anatomic factors that influence the prognosis of furcation involvement.

b. Enumerate the acute gingival infections. What are the signs and symptoms of acute necrotising ulcerative

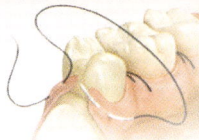

9   PATTERN PAPER

SECTION – B

(10 × 2 = 20)

❏ **Answer the following:**

a. Acute periodontal abscess.

b. Trauma from occlusion.

c. Gingival crevicular fluid.

d. Chronic desquamative gingivitis and its treatment.

e. Principles of instrumentation.

f. Epulis.

g. Local drug delivery.

h. Oral physiotherapy.

i. Refractory periodontitis.

j. Microscopic picture of gingiva.

SECTION – C

(2 × 10 = 20)

❏ **Write long answer:**

a. Classify gingival enlargements. Discuss drug-induced gingival enlargements for their clinical features, in detail and treatment of dilantin-induced gingival enlargement.

b. Define prognosis. Enumerate only factors considered to determine individual and overall prognosis of periodontically diseased dentition, and discuss in detail the factors considered in prognosis of individual teeth.

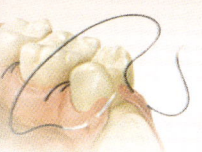
PATTERN PAPER 10

SECTION – B

(10 × 2 = 20)

❏ **Write short answers:**

a. Enumerate the factors of prognosis of individual tooth in periodontal diseases.

b. Classify periodontal diseases.

c. Mention about macroscopic and microscopic structures of normal gingiva.

d. Describe the relationship between diabetes and periodontitis.

e. Theories of calculus formation.

f. Treatment of ANUG.

g. Methods of pocket elimination.

h. Advances in periodontal probing.

i. Tooth mobility.

j. Peri-implantitis

SECTION – C

(2 × 10 = 20)

❏ **Write long answer:**

a. What is oral physiotherapy? Describe the indication contraindication, advantage and disadvantages of modified Stilman's method.

b. Discuss the causes of gingival bleeding. How will you proceed to investigate such case?

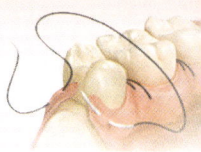

11 PATTERN PAPER

SECTION – B

(10 × 2 = 20)

❑ **Answer the following:**

a. Mention the importance of cementum in periodontal therapy.

b. Enumerate the interdental aids.

c. Treatment of acute pericoronitis.

d. Pathologic migration.

e. Defence mechanism of gingiva.

f. Composition of calculus.

g. Furcation involvement.

h. ENAP.

i. Peri-implantitis.

j. Hypersensitivity.

SECTION – C

(2 × 10 = 20)

❑ **Write long answer:**

a. How will you prepare the patient for periodontal surgery? Discuss in detail the common general consideration to carry out various periodontal surgical procedures.

b. Classify gingival enlargement and write in detail on drug-induced gingival enlargement.

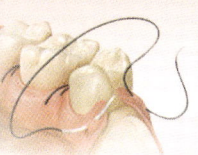

PATTERN PAPER 12

SECTION – B

(10 × 2 = 20)

❏ **Answer the following**:

a. Bone destruction patterns in periodontal disease.

b. Refractory periodontitis.

c. Theories of mineralization of calculus.

d. Phases of periodontal therapy.

e. Periodontal abscess vs. periapical abscess.

f. Consistancy of gingiva.

g. Sharpening of periodontal instruments.

h. Iatrogenic factors.

i. Bone graft materials.

j. Excisional new attachment procedure (ENAP)

SECTION – C

(2 × 10 = 20)

❏ **Write long answer:**

a. Define plaque. Describe the classification, composition, structure and formation of dental plaque in detail.

b. Define mucogingival surgery. Give the classification and indications of it. Describe the free gingival autograft technique for gingival augmentation apical to recession in detail.

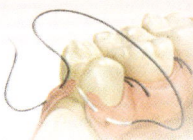

13   PATTERN PAPER

SECTION – B

(10 × 2 = 20)

❑ **Answer the following:**

a. Specific plaque hypothesis.

b. Periotron.

c. Bone blend.

d. BANA.

e. Indications for root resection.

f. Laboratory investigations of acute herpetic gingivo-stomatitis.

g. Differentiate between gingivectomy and gingivoplasty.

h. Differentiate between suprabony and infrabony pockets.

i. Differentiate between area-specific and universal curettes.

j. Enumerate various controlled release local drug delivery system.

SECTION – C

(2 × 10 = 20)

❑ **Write long answer:**

a. Define flap. Classify basic flap. Give a step by step accout of modified Widman flap.

b. Define periodontal ligament. Describe in detail the functions of periodontal ligament.

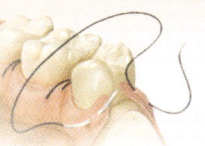

PATTERN PAPER   14

SECTION – B

(10 × 2 = 20)

❑ **Answer the following:**

a. Gingival blood supply and innervation.

b. Possible role of ascorbic acid deficiency in etiology of periodontal disease.

c. Changes in root surface wall of periodontal pockets.

d. Causes of and changes produced by primary trauma from occlusion.

e. Periodontal manifestations of leukaemia.

f. Role of tooth morphology in assessing prognosis of individual tooth.

g. Instrument stabilization.

h. Controlled-release local delivery system.

i. Indications of coronoplasty and enumerate steps of coronoplasty.

j. Indications and side effects of chlorhexidine.

SECTION – C

(2 × 10 = 20)

❑ **Write long answer:**

a. Enumerate acute gingival lesions. Discuss in detail etiology, clinical features, histopathology and differential diagnosis of acute herpetic gingivostomatitis.

b. Describe non-graft associated reconstructive periodontal surgical techniques.

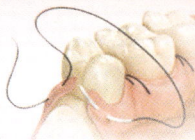

15   PATTERN PAPER

SECTION – B

(10 × 2 = 20)

❑ **Write short answers to the following:**

a. Definition and functions of gingival fibers.

b. Describe in short oral manifestations of scurvy.

c. Define and give the etiology of halitosis.

d. Sequelae of food impaction.

e. Commercial allografts.

f. Periodontal splints.

g. Refractory periodontitis.

h. Clinical and radiological changes in trauma from occlusion.

i. Interdental cleanser in type II embrasures.

j. Give definition and factors influencing individual prognosis of periodontal disease.

SECTION – C

(2 × 10 = 20)

❑ **Write long answer:**

a. Define, give broad classification and composition of dental plaque. Describe the characteristics of the gel-like matrix of biofilm.

b. Describe various aspects of gingivectomy surgery.

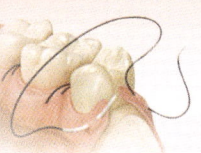

PATTERN PAPER 16

SECTION – B

(10 × 2 = 20)

❑ **Answer the following:**
a. Define furcation involvement and give its classification.
b. What is gingival col? What is its significance?
c. What are the causes of tooth mobility?
d. What is subgingival plaque? Give its classification.
e. What is the treatment of acute herpetic gingivos-tomatitis?
f. Define mucogingival surgery and enumerate various mucogingival surgical procedures.
g. Primary and secondary trauma from occlusion.
h. Define prognosis. Enumerate factors to consider when determining a prognosis.
i. Fenestration and dehiscence.
j. Enumerate the principles of sharpening of instruments.

SECTION – C

(2 × 10 = 20)

❑ **Write long answer:**
a. Define gingiva. Describe the clinical and microscopic features of normal healthy gingiva.
b. Define osseous surgery. Describe the osseous resection technique in detail.

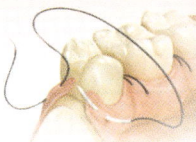

17 PATTERN PAPER

SECTION - B

(10 × 2 = 20)

❑ **Answer the following:**

a. Give the etiology, difference and treatment of gingival and periodontal abscess.

b. Microscopic features of healthy gingiva.

c. Describe in short the important factors to prevent recurrence of periodontal disease.

d. Describe in short the various methods of obtaining bone graft from intraoral sites.

e. What is adaptive remodelling of the periodontium in response to external force?

f. Acute episodes of gingival bleeding.

g. Hypercementosis.

h. Pathological migration of teeth.

i. Indications of mucogingival surgery.

j. Gingival crevicular fluid

SECTION - C

(2 × 10 = 20)

❑ **Write long answer:**

a. Define and give classification of periodontal flap. What are objective and essential step of "Modified Widman Flap"?

b. Define gingival recession. Difference with diagram the type of recession. Enumerate the etiology of recession and describe the procedure of lateral sliding flap

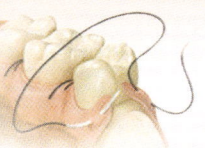
PATTERN PAPER 18

SECTION – B

(10 × 2 = 30)

❑ **Write short answer to the following:**

a. What are the various indications for hospital periodontal surgery?

b. State the composition of dental calculus

c. What is halitosis?

d. Buttressing bone formation

e. Juvenile periodontitis

f. Pregnancy tumour

g. Define and classify dental plaque

h. Describe in short the various osseous defects seen in periodontal diseases

i. Define occlusal adjustment. Mention the various procedures by which it is achieved

j. Explain with diagrams the pathways of spread of inflammation

SECTION – C

(2 × 10 = 20)

❑ **Write long answer to each of the following:**

a. State the systemic conditions modifying the clinical appearance of periodontal tissue. Describe in detail the clinical features of any three such conditions.

b. Define pocket. Give its classification and describe various methods of pocket elimination.

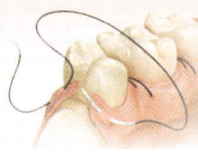

19 | PATTERN PAPER

SECTION – B

(10 × 2 = 20)

❑ **Answer the following:**

   a. Gingival crevicular fluid

   b. Dental calculus.

   c. Food impaction.

   d. Traumatic occlusion.

   e. Corelation of clinical and histopathological features of periodontal pocket.

   f. Osseous defects.

   g. Toothbrush.

   h. Acute pericoronitis.

   i. Chronic desquamative gingivitis.

   j. Indication of flap operation.

SECTION – C

(2 × 10 = 20)

❑ **Write long answer:**

   a. Define prognosis. Discuss the factors considered for prognosis of periodontal involved case.

   b. Classify gingival enlargement. Discuss in detail signs, symptoms and treatment of dilantin sodium gingival enlargement.

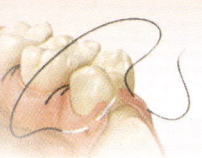

PATTERN PAPER 20

SECTION – B

(10 × 2 = 20)

❑ **Answer the following:**

a. Give Millers classification of gingival recession.

b. Enumerate various theories of mineralization of calculus.

c. Enumerate the different means of taking a gingivectomy incision.

d. Define coronoplasty. What are its indications?

e. What are the various causes of increased tooth mobility?

f. Enumerate the protective component of saliva in periodontal disease process.

g. Define periodontology and periodontics.

h. Define periodontium. What does it comprise of?

i. Define trauma from occlusion. What are the various stages of tissue response in trauma from occlusion?

j. What are the indications for gingival curettage?

SECTION – C

(2 × 10 = 20)

❑ **Write long answers on the following:**

a. Discuss in detail the functions of the periodontal ligament.

b. Classify bony defects in periodontal disease. How would you establish the prognosis of such defects?

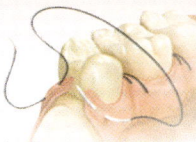

21   PATTERN PAPER

SECTION – B

(10 × 2 = 20)

❑ **Answer the following:**

 a. HIV and the periodontium.

 b. Guided tissue regeneration.

 c. Dentifrices.

 d. Treatment of periodontal abscess.

 e. What are the guidelines for preparing a splint?

 f. What are the principles of sharpening periodontal instruments?

 g. What are the uses of radiography in periodontal therapy?

 h. What are the causes of failure of gingivectomy?

 i. What is the difference between a gingival abscess and a periodontal abscess?

 j. Classify periodontal pockets.

SECTION – C

(2 × 10 = 20)

❑ **Write long answers on the following:**

 a. Define gingiva. What are the parts of the normal gingiva? Describe the microscopic picture of normal gingiva.

 b. Define prognosis. What factors will you take into consideration when determining the prognosis of a case?

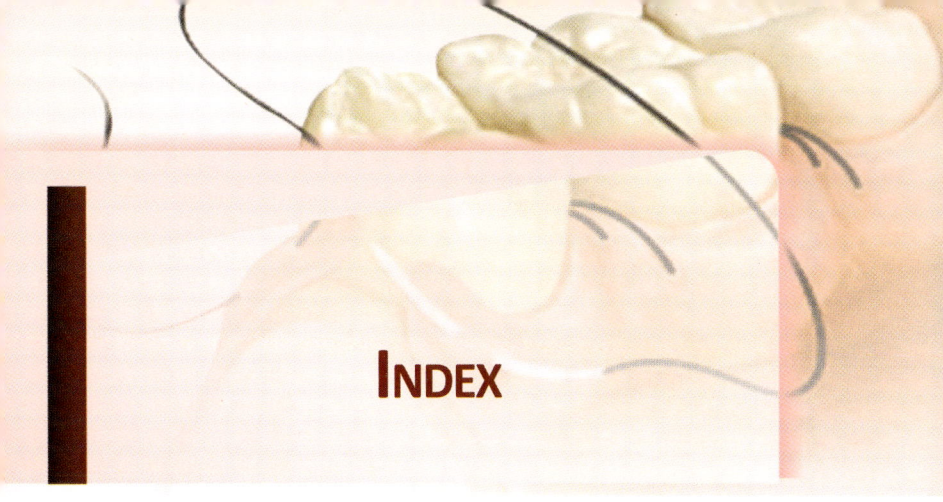

INDEX

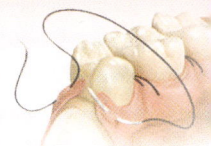

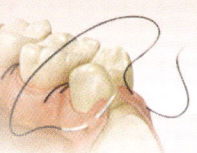

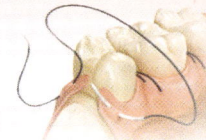

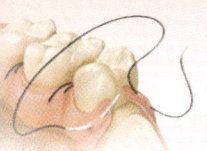

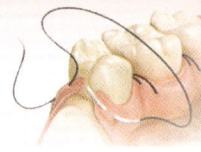

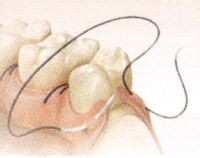

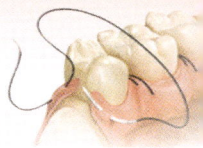